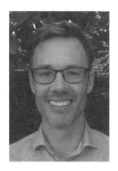

Dr Kailas Roberts is a consultant psychiatrist and psychogeriatrician with over ten years' experience in the field of old-age psychiatry. He runs a busy private practice caring for people with cognitive difficulties, and advises on management of the behavioural and psychological difficulties that often accompany dementia. He lives in Brisbane, and this is his first book.

yourbraininmind.com

T0308899

Mind Your Brain

The Essential Australian Guide to Dementia

DR KAILAS ROBERTS

First published 2021 by University of Queensland Press
PO Box 6042, St Lucia, Queensland 4067 Australia

uqp.com.au
reception@uqp.com.au

Cover design by Christabella Designs
Typeset in 12/15 pt Bembo Std by Post Pre-press Group, Brisbane
Printed in Australia by McPherson's Printing Group

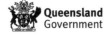 The University of Queensland Press is supported by the Queensland
Government through Arts Queensland.

 The University of Queensland Press is assisted by the
Australian Government through the Australia Council, its
arts funding and advisory body.

A catalogue record for this book is available from the National Library of Australia

ISBN 978 0 7022 6309 5 (pbk)
ISBN 978 0 7022 6468 9 (epdf)
ISBN 978 0 7022 6469 6 (epub)
ISBN 978 0 7022 6470 2 (kindle)

University of Queensland Press uses papers that are natural, renewable and recyclable products
made from wood grown in well-managed forests and other controlled sources. The logging and
manufacturing processes conform to the environmental regulations of the country of origin.

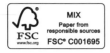

To Jennie, for pointing me in the right direction and holding the fort.

Contents

Introduction

In Australia, over 400,000 people are known to have dementia. This number is projected to increase massively over the coming years and decades, as we are living longer than ever before. Globally, the numbers are even more mind-boggling: 50 million people are known to have the condition, and it is estimated that by 2050 this figure will have trebled.

At its heart, though, the experience of dementia is a profoundly personal one, not only for the person with the condition, but also for the many others around them – family, friends and other carers. The condition can throw lives into chaos and force us to make big changes and difficult decisions. For these reasons, and because it is a condition we cannot cure, there is a preponderance of negative emotions associated with dementia – anxiety and stress, pessimism, despondency and sometimes even despair.

Yet humans have a remarkable capacity to adapt to difficult circumstances, and I have frequently been impressed by how well patients of mine cope when dementia is confirmed. My experience as a medical specialist in the field of memory loss and dementia suggests there are several critical factors in coping successfully. These include:

- Knowing all you can about the condition
- Knowing that you arc doing all you can to help
- Feeling competent to face the challenges that arise
- Knowing when and how to access support.

If you are a carer, looking after yourself as well as the person you are caring for is also vital.

Mind Your Brain aims to provide advice on all the key issues related to dementia. Many patients and carers I have worked with have started out with little understanding of these issues, some of which are fundamental. This is reflected in the questions I am frequently asked:

- How can I protect myself against memory loss and dementia?
- What even is dementia? Are Alzheimer's and dementia the same thing?
- What are the symptoms of the condition and how does it progress?
- How long will I live once I have the condition?
- What else might be causing my problems with thinking? Could it be reversible?
- How can I best help someone who is experiencing dementia?

My experience has also shown me there is an abundance of myths concerning the condition, including:

- That we will all get dementia in the end
- That if you don't have memory loss, you don't have dementia
- That if someone in your family develops dementia, you will get it too
- That there's nothing you can do about dementia, so there's no point being assessed for it.

My goal in writing this book is to empower those experiencing dementia and those caring for them with knowledge and advice. It will also be of value to those concerned they might develop dementia in the future. Once you know what you are dealing with, it is easier to make plans and manage the situation.

The information contained within this book comes, in the main, from three sources: first, my informed reading of the vast and increasing literature on the topic (there is a wealth of research available online that ensures clinicians are up to date and making evidence-based decisions); second, regular discussions with my medical and allied health colleagues, many of whom have given me invaluable advice over the years; finally, and of equal importance, the conversations I have had with those experiencing dementia, as well as with their carers and loved ones. I have learnt much from them – how they have managed to cope, what has worked and what hasn't, what their biggest fears are, what they really want to know, and what help they need. I hope that sharing this knowledge through this book will make the journey of dementia easier for those embarking upon it.

The message implicit in this book is that there is hope. Yes, there are some inescapable and unpalatable truths – dementia is permanent and, on the whole, gets worse with time – but there is much that can be done to reduce the risk of developing dementia, to delay its onset, and to make the journey easier once it is established. It is not all doom and gloom. Many individuals (and their loved ones) can enjoy long periods of contentment and a good quality of life despite the progressive nature of the condition. There are ways to improve memory and other cognitive skills in dementia, or at least to make the most of what we have. Likewise, there are treatments available to manage the physical and psychological symptoms that frequently accompany the condition. To avoid unnecessary suffering, it is critical to be informed about these matters.

My intention with this book is to spread this message of hope, and to provide practical tips for the person experiencing dementia as well as those involved in their care. Of course, dementia is a medical illness, and so its confirmation involves consultation with medical professionals, whether that be the local family doctor or a specialist. Importantly, this book is not intended to replace that process, but to augment it – to help you understand the approach that is taken, and to guide conversations that you may have with your doctor.

Although this book is written from an Australian perspective, and some of the advice relating to legal issues, respite and residential care will differ from country to country, I have tried to ensure that it is as universally applicable as possible, and that the large majority of the information it contains is relevant wherever in the world the reader may be.

How to use this book

The structure of this book recognises that different readers will come to it with different needs and goals, so I have endeavoured to make it as user-friendly as possible. The book therefore has two main parts.

Part One explores the science of dementia: how the healthy brain functions, how it changes as we age, the causes of cognitive decline and how to prevent it, and what dementia actually is. It also describes the main types of dementia: Alzheimer's disease, vascular dementia, frontotemporal dementia, alcohol-related dementia and forms of predominantly subcortical dementia.

Part Two focuses on the lived experience of dementia, in all its aspects: being assessed and diagnosed, the symptoms of the disease and treatments for them, the physical and psychological challenges dementia can pose, as well as practical life changes that can maximise individuals' comfort and happiness. It discusses legal and ethical issues around dementia, residential care options, and dying and end-of-life care. This section of the book also explores how to manage as a carer. Although looking after someone with dementia can be difficult and distressing, much can be done to make the situation easier.

The appendices offer further information about organisations, websites and other resources that may be of value to those with dementia or those caring for them.

PART ONE

Understanding Dementia

SECTION I
The Healthy Brain

1

How the Brain Functions

- The brain consists of many billions of nerve cells that interact with each other via electrical and chemical messages.

- The brain can be divided into two halves, each containing four lobes with different but overlapping functions. These make up the cortex of the brain.

- Deeper in the brain are subcortical structures that influence movement, emotions and certain types of memory. Some parts of the subcortex also function as our life-support system.

- Dementia can affect any of the structures of the brain, whether cortical or subcortical.

- The brain is responsible for our cognitive abilities – processes that allow us to understand and manipulate ourselves and our environment. Cognitive functions include attention, memory, orientation, language, calculation, praxis, gnosis, visuospatial skills and executive abilities. All may be affected by dementia.

The brain is responsible for all that we do, and arguably all that we are. It controls human functions as basic as breathing, movement and sensation, and is critical for the optimal performance of all our bodily systems, such as those involving the heart, hormones and the gut. On a more profound level, our brain allows us to think, and to interact with the world and people around us. It is responsible for creating our sense of who we are.

Of course, as with all other parts of the body, aspects of normal brain function can go wrong. Unless we know how something is supposed to work, it is impossible to tell why things malfunction. This is as true for something as complex as the human brain as it is for something far simpler, such as the engine of a car. It may be obvious that something is not right – the car does not start, or we cannot recall what we have done in the recent past – but unless we know how the different components of each system contribute to the overall function, we can only guess at the source of the problem.

This chapter explains how the brain's various parts operate and interact with each other. (It is easy to get lost in the rabbit hole of neuroanatomy and neurophysiology, though, so I have kept the discussion relatively simple.) It also summarises the skills enabled by the brain that allow us to function within our complex physical and social environment. It is the degradation of these *cognitive skills* that underpins the problems we see in dementia.

A mass of circuitry

The brain weighs, on average, 1.3 to 1.4 kilograms, slightly more in males. This equates generally to about 2 per cent of our body weight, though it is so active it uses 20 to 30 per cent of our energy needs. It is made up of billions of nerve cells. Some of these are directly responsible for transmitting messages throughout the brain and are known as *neurons*. These cells are all connected to each other in a vast circuit. It has been estimated that there are more neuronal connections in the brain than there are stars in our galaxy. The other type of nerve cells are called *glia* (or *glial cells*). These play more of a supportive role for the neurons and do not send messages themselves.

In order for the brain to perform its role in the impressively efficient way it does, it needs to send messages both within its own circuitry and to other parts of the body. For this to happen, messages need to travel from one end of a nerve cell to the other, and then onward to other cells nearby.

Within an individual nerve cell, messages are conveyed from the cell *body*, along a fine, fingery outgrowth called an *axon*, to the other end. The axon can be very long – sometimes over a metre. The message at this stage is in the form of an electrical signal, and the axon is insulated by a material called *myelin* to prevent the messages being discharged elsewhere (much like the insulating plastic around an electrical wire). Once along the axon, the electrical signal is conveyed to a number of structures called *axon terminals*.

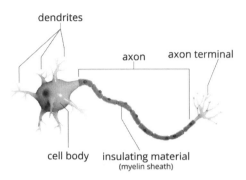

A neuron: electrical messages travel from one end to the other.

From the axon terminals, messages are carried to other nearby nerve cells in the form of chemicals called *neurotransmitters*. The chemicals are released from the terminals and travel across a gap between the nerve cells known as a *synapse*. On the other side, they are received by smaller outgrowths on adjacent cells called *dendrites*, which are directly connected to the body of this receiving nerve cell. If the nerve cell were a tree, the dendrites would be its roots. The messages may be received by multiple nerve cells at once; in this way, they are spread efficiently throughout the neuronal circuitry of the brain.

Brain anatomy

Grey and white matter

If you were to cut a brain into sections, you would see that various parts are coloured differently. These shades correspond to the different parts of the neurons. The body, dendrites and axon terminals have a pinkish grey colour, and are therefore known as *grey matter*. The axons look pinkish white and are known as *white matter*. The white matter is in some ways like a subway that connects stations (the bodies). Damage to the brain can occur in both the grey and white matter, and messages can be interrupted in either situation.

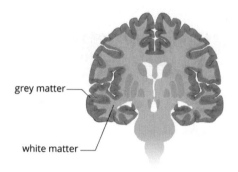

The brain consists of grey and white matter, each housing different parts of the nerve cell.

The cortex

The wrinkly outermost part of the brain that we all recognise is known as the *cortex*. This is composed of grey matter, and is between 2 and 4 millimetres thick. It is like a thin cloak wrapped around the deeper parts of the brain. Structures within this part of the brain are referred to as *cortical*.

The cortex can be divided into two halves, or *hemispheres*, left and right. They are joined by a thick bundle of nerve fibres known as the *corpus callosum*, allowing one side to communicate with the other. Damage to one side of our brain tends to produce movement problems with our limbs on the opposite side. We are increasingly recognising that one hemisphere can also compensate for damage to the other. Each side may have differing functions to a degree, though. For instance, the left hemisphere is probably more relevant for language. It is also the dominant hemisphere for 90 per cent of people, accounting for the fact that most of us have better control of our right hand.

Each hemisphere contains four *lobes*, or sections. These are the *frontal lobe*, the *temporal lobe*, the *parietal lobe* and the *occipital lobe*. Each of these has a number of different functions.

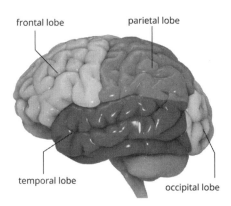

frontal lobe

parietal lobe

temporal lobe

occipital lobe

Each half of the brain has four lobes.

If the brain were an orchestra, the *frontal lobe* would be the conductor. It regulates and oversees many of the other processes in the brain, allowing us to use reason and make sound decisions about what we are doing. It is responsible for our *executive skills*, which help us complete more complex thinking tasks to better plan and organise ourselves. Accurate expression of language is governed by the frontal lobe. The frontal lobe is also important in helping us notice things in our environment and keeping information 'in mind' for short periods – such as remembering a phone number that has been given to us so we can use it soon after. This is known as *working memory*. The frontal lobe also allows us to retrieve our long-term memories, which are stored in other parts of our brain. The foremost part of the frontal lobe is called the *prefrontal cortex*, and may have especial relevance for our executive abilities and attention. In many ways, the frontal lobe is what makes us human: it enables us to choose not to act on our basic impulses, and to instead engage in socially appropriate behaviour.

The *temporal lobe* is critical for memory formation, as well as for distributing these memories to other parts of the brain, where they become long-term memories. Knowing where we are (orientation) is also reliant on this lobe. A small structure in the temporal lobe, the *hippocampus*, is of particular relevance to memory function. It is often damaged early in Alzheimer's disease, the most common cause of dementia. This lobe is also important for interpreting sounds, including speech, and for making sense of what we see.

The *parietal lobe* allows us to know where various parts of our body are in space, and to understand where other objects are in relation to us – so-called *visuospatial skills*. It plays an important role in purposeful movement, a process known as *praxis*, which allows us to complete many everyday tasks. The parietal lobe is also important for our language function, our ability to perform mathematics and our ability to recognise objects through touch.

The *occipital lobe*, the smallest of the four, allows us to interpret and understand what our eyes are seeing.

It is important to understand that dementia can affect any of the lobes of the brain, and cause impairment to any of the associated skills. Memory loss – the symptom most people think of in relation to dementia – is only one of a number of problems that may develop.

Beneath the cortex

The deeper parts of the brain are collectively known as the *subcortex*, and structures within them are often referred to as *subcortical*. The subcortical structures can be affected by dementia, sometimes before the cortical structures. Examples of subcortical structures include:

- The *cerebellum*, which is critical for balance and movement (especially fine movement). It is particularly prone to the effects of alcohol, which is why one can become unbalanced when under the influence. The cerebellum may also have some role in regulating our emotions.
- The *brainstem*, which connects the brain with the spinal cord. It contains a number of other structures, including the *pons*, the *midbrain*, and the *medulla oblongata*. The brainstem is critical for basic bodily functions such as swallowing, breathing and facial movements. It is like our life-support system. Even small areas of damage (*lesions*) in the brainstem can cause profound changes, such as breathing disorders, and problems with swallowing and speech.

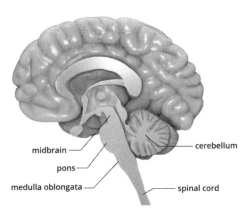

The location of the brainstem (midbrain, pons and medulla oblongata) and cerebellum.

- The *basal ganglia*, a group of small structures (known as *nuclei*) deep within the brain. They are thought to have numerous roles, including regulation of movement, integration of memory and maintenance of attention. Parkinson's disease may be caused by damage to the basal ganglia. Psychiatric symptoms such as mood changes, delusions and hallucinations, and anxiety can occur with damage to the basal ganglia.
- The *limbic system*, a set of connected zones of tissue (nuclei again) that lie immediately below the inside portion of the temporal lobe. Some of these are subcortical, such as the *amygdala*. This almond-shaped structure attaches an emotional significance to a memory (such as joy, shame or guilt). These memories seem especially immune to degradation. The amygdala also plays a pivotal role in fear, an emotion that is especially potent when it comes to memory formation. Other limbic structures, such as the hippocampus (mentioned earlier) are actually cortical structures. The *thalamus* relays motor (movement) and sensory signals to the cerebral cortex. The *hypothalamus* maintains the balance of numerous vital functions, regulating temperature, sleep and appetite, for example. The limbic system more generally plays a significant role in our emotional state, motivation and long-term memory storage.

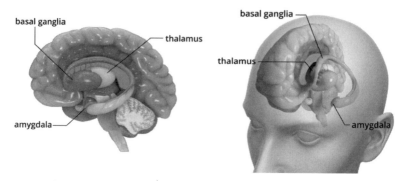

Location of parts of the limbic system and the basal ganglia.

When dementia affects these subcortical structures, the symptoms may be quite different to when the cortical areas are damaged. The most obvious initial problems may be with movement, balance, emotions or other bodily functions. As it progresses, dementia often affects both cortical and subcortical regions, leading to a mix of symptoms, becoming more 'global' in effect.

The ventricles

The other structures worth noting in discussions around dementia are the *ventricles*, which are cavities that run throughout the brain. They are filled with *cerebrospinal fluid*, which bathes and protects the brain and the spinal cord. Enlargement of the ventricles can occur in conditions where the brain shrinks, including Alzheimer's disease. Sometimes, the ventricular enlargement itself causes problems. This is known as *hydrocephalus* and is discussed in Chapter 9.

Cognitive skills

Cognition is often defined as 'a mental process of acquiring knowledge and understanding through thought, experience and the senses'. When discussing dementia, however, it is more helpful to consider cognition as 'our capacity to competently adapt to the environment around us'. Without adequate cognition, we may be unable to accurately process or use the various stimuli – things we see, hear or otherwise experience – that our environment creates. We may then lose awareness of where we are, why we are there, what we are doing, who and what is around us, and how we should react.

Skills related to cognition are known as *cognitive skills*. These include *attention, memory function, orientation, language function, calculation, visuospatial skills, gnosis, praxis* and *executive abilities*. All of these may be impaired in different forms of dementia.

Let's look at each of these in a little more detail.

Attention

Attention refers to our ability to notice or highlight things in our environment. We *pay attention* to numerous stimuli, including what we see and hear. Without attention, we do not consciously register what is happening around us and therefore there is nothing to later remember. Attention is divided into various parts: *selective attention* (when we focus on one thing among a number of things), *divided attention* (when we focus on more than one thing at once, such as talking while we walk), and *sustained attention* (when we remain focused on one thing for a while – closely related to concentration).

Two areas of the brain are thought to be particularly important in regulating attention. One is the *prefrontal cortex*, which is the foremost part of the frontal lobe. If we are deliberately trying to pay attention to something – such as when reading a book – the prefrontal cortex is responsible. The other is the parietal lobe, which is involved when our attention is suddenly drawn to something unexpected – hearing someone scream, for instance.

Memory function

Memory is our ability to remember information that comes to us in the form of *stimuli* – messages from our environment, whether in the form of pictures, sounds or other senses. Memory function can be divided into *sensory memory, short-term memory* and *long-term memory*. Different parts of the brain may be responsible for each.

Sensory memory is the shortest type of memory and is really just a mental representation of what we sense (see, hear, feel, smell and so on). A very brief mental image of a car that has just passed by is an example of sensory memory.

Short-term memory, often used interchangeably with the term *working memory*, is the part of our memory in which we hold information for short periods so that we can manipulate it. Examples include following the elements of a conversation so that we can respond appropriately, and mentally reciting the items on a shopping list when we enter a supermarket. This type of memory only stays with us as long as we are consciously thinking about it, and usually lasts no longer than a minute.

For our memory to be recalled at a later date (after it has left our conscious awareness for the first time), it needs to become encoded by the hippocampus. This structure acts like a sorting centre, receiving short-term memories and distributing them to different parts of the cortex where they become *long-term memories*. We then have *acquired* these memories for future remembering – a process formally known as *acquisition*.

There are two types of long-term memory. One is called *explicit memory*, and relates to things that have happened to us (episodic memory) or knowledge we have learnt over our lives (semantic memory). The frontal lobe is employed to *retrieve* such memories – that is, to remember them and bring them to our attention again. This process is known formally as *retrieval*. The other type of long-term memory is termed *implicit*. These are our 'autopilot' memories – ones we don't consciously remember, such as how to drive a car or ride a bike. Explicit and implicit memories are stored in different areas – the first in the cortex and the second in subcortical structures like the cerebellum and basal ganglia – which is why we may be unable to recall a recent event but still be able to drive a car.

Orientation

Orientation is our ability to know where we are, in both space and time – referred to as *spatial* and *temporal orientation*, respectively. If we cannot orient ourselves, we are *disoriented*. This cognitive skill involves a variety of different areas of the brain, including the frontal, temporal and parietal lobes.

Language function

This skill relates both to our ability to express what we want to in speech, and to understand what is being said to us. It is also important for written comprehension and expression. Although a number of areas of the brain may be necessary for this skill, the frontal and parietal/temporal lobes seem particularly important for producing speech and understanding speech, respectively. When an individual has difficulties with spoken language (despite the fact that the muscles governing speech are intact) they are described as being *aphasic* or *dysphasic*.

Calculation

This skill allows us to perform basic math operations such as addition, subtraction, division and multiplication. The inability to calculate – or *acalculia* – is classically related to parietal lobe dysfunction, though it can also occur after damage to the frontal lobe.

Visuospatial abilities

These skills allow us to understand what we see around us, and our relationship in space to other objects in our environment, such as how far away something may be. They allow us to accurately perceive depth, a vital skill in navigating objects such as stairs and in facilitating other daily tasks – getting in and out of a bath, for example, or sitting down on a chair. Feeding ourselves can be a challenge without adequate visuospatial skills, while even mild impairment of visuospatial abilities means driving may become unsafe.

Visuospatial skills also allow us to know our environment; without them we may not recognise even familiar routes and locations.

The circuitry that allows us to use our visuospatial skills is widely distributed through the brain, including in the occipital, parietal and temporal lobes.

Gnosis

This skill allows us to recognise people and objects that should be familiar. There are a number of subtypes depending on the sense involved. Problems recognising what we see is termed *visual agnosia*.

Faulty recognition of sound, including speech, is termed *auditory agnosia*. Being unable to recognise by touch is called *tactile agnosia*.

Praxis

This skill allows us to voluntarily move various parts of our body. It is critical for us to perform everyday functions such as getting dressed, manipulating objects (to brush our teeth, for example) and walking in a coordinated fashion. The circuitry involves the frontal and parietal lobes, as well as subcortical structures such as the basal ganglia. When someone has difficulties with these tasks, we refer to this as *apraxia*.

Executive skills

In many ways, it is our executive abilities that differentiate humans from most other species. They allow us to plan ahead, organise ourselves, sustain our motivation and stay focused, and they stop us from acting on unhelpful impulses. They underpin our ability to work together, be socially appropriate and self-regulate. The ability to switch from one way of thinking to another – *mental flexibility* – is related to executive function. Working memory is also considered an executive skill.

All these abilities rely heavily on the frontal lobe, although damage to subcortical structures can also cause impairment.

2

Normal Ageing and Cognition

- Normal ageing results in some cognitive changes, but not everyone will get dementia.
- Age-related cognitive changes should not cause significant impairment of daily functioning.
- The brain shrinks as we get older and often accumulates damage from impaired blood supply. These processes do not always result in dementia, though are often present on brain scans.
- Cognitive changes associated with ageing include slowing of thinking, mild word-finding difficulties, problems with acquiring new memories, mild problems holding information 'in mind' for short periods, and executive changes.
- Language function, practical skills that are well learnt, visuospatial skills, and general knowledge are not impaired greatly by normal ageing.

It is an unfortunate fact, and one I recognise in myself, that age is not necessarily kind to the brain. We often feel less 'sharp' and words don't come as easily. We compensate for our degrading memory by using lists and diaries more enthusiastically. Our speed of thinking and response times seem to slow. This is unlikely to be a figment of our imagination, as the evidence does suggest a deterioration in some cognitive skills as we go through life – perhaps starting as early as our thirties. On the whole, though, normal brain ageing should not significantly affect our day-to-day life. We find ways around the changes.

I am often asked to see patients who are worried about a decline in their memory and conclude that their difficulties are just the product of healthy ageing. Conversely, I have also seen many individuals who wrongly assume their marked deterioration in memory and thinking skills is simply part of being old. I worry more about the second group, of course, especially as I often don't see them until their dementia is quite advanced, and we know that treatments for dementia are better started when it is in its mild stages.

This chapter aims to provide information on how to tell the difference between normal cognitive ageing and other, more problematic conditions. Although I would always advise individuals with progressive and enduring cognitive changes to speak with their GP about their concerns, there are certain red flags that should not be ignored.

Changes in brain structure with age

As we age, our brain shrinks. This begins sooner than most of us would imagine, possibly as early as our third or fourth decade of life. If we are healthy, the rate of shrinkage – or *atrophy* as it is also known – tends to be relatively slow until our sixties or seventies, when it starts to accelerate.

Shrinkage in the brain occurs in the grey matter, leading to a thinning of the cortex. Areas that seem especially susceptible to this shrinkage include the prefrontal cortex and the temporal lobes. Reduced volume in these areas is also typical of pathological processes such as Alzheimer's disease or frontotemporal dementia. In these latter conditions, however, the shrinkage occurs more rapidly and may be considerably more severe.

White matter also undergoes changes with age. As white matter is formed from the insulated parts of the nerve cell that carry messages from one end to the other, it is not surprising that damage to this area may lead to a reduction in the ability of the nerve cells to transmit messages – which in turn can negatively impact memory and other cognitive functions.

Scans of the brain, such as CT scans and MRI scans, can be used to assess the degree and location of shrinkage, though this is only part of the puzzle. To make the clinical interpretation more difficult, some individuals with considerably more shrinkage than age alone would cause do not have any obvious cognitive problems. Equally, others may be experiencing many of the clinical symptoms of dementia and yet show minimal brain shrinkage. Because of this considerable individual variation, it is helpful to have previous scans – say, from ten or twenty years prior – with which to compare the new scans, but this is not something doctors usually have access to.

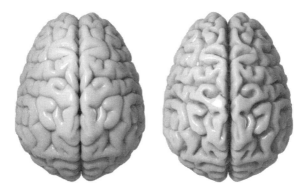

Young brain (left) vs old brain; note the shrunken appearance of the aged brain.

The age-related shrinkage we see is in part due to the death of the nerve cells. Interestingly, some of this death may be due to the toxic effects of a protein called *beta-amyloid*, the accumulation of which is one of the core problems in Alzheimer's disease. It has been estimated that beta-amyloid occurs in up to 30 per cent of the brains of normal healthy adults, and although its presence alone does not indicate dementia is present, there is speculation that it may signal an individual is at higher risk of developing the condition over time. A reduction in the size of the nerve cells and the number of connections between them – phenomena that occur naturally with age – also contributes to grey matter loss and cognitive change.

The ability of the bloodstream to provide adequate nutrients to the brain also diminishes with age. This may be related in part to *inflammation* and *oxidative stress* (a concept we'll explore in Chapter 8, on Alzheimer's disease). Conditions like *atherosclerosis*, where fatty plaques may coat the inside of blood vessels, can also narrow these vessels and reduce blood flow. The elasticity of the vessel walls also lessens, meaning they are less able to tolerate changes in blood pressure; this increases the likelihood of tiny strokes occurring in the surrounding brain tissue.

As with shrinkage, problems with blood supply as we age, which manifest as small or large strokes, can be visualised on brain scans, though, again, someone can be relatively symptom-free despite significant damage on the scan.

How age affects our ability to think

One of the key distinctions between the cognitive deterioration associated with normal ageing and that of dementia is the extent of loss of function. Changes associated with age alone do not explain a situation where an individual is unable to perform their day-to-day activities – or *activities of daily living*, as they are often called. These activities are myriad, and include washing, dressing, cooking, shopping, paying bills and remembering appointments.

The cognitive changes that occur with ageing also tend to occur over a very long time frame – years or even decades. A considerably more rapid decline should be a red flag that something else may be occurring.

The most noticeable change with ageing is that of *cognitive slowing*. It is usual for the elderly to take longer to think things through, to process information and to come up with answers for problems. Given time, however, they should generally be expected to come up with accurate answers. In addition, the specific ability to find the right word in conversation tends to decline with age. This leads to more 'tip of the tongue' moments than we experience in our younger years.

There is also some deterioration in the ability to form new memories, and in working memory. This may be due to a deterioration in attention or in the ability to filter out irrelevant stimuli. Someone who is older may not remember all the details of a recent event – although they will remember some. By contrast, someone experiencing dementia may not recall the event even occurring. Our memory for things that have happened in our lives – our *episodic memory* – tends to be affected earlier than our store of factual knowledge – our *semantic memory*.

Certain executive abilities also undergo age-related changes. For example, we experience a reduction in mental flexibility, and in our capacity to inhibit inappropriate responses. Executive skills with a timed component involving movement are especially susceptible to the effects of age – probably due to reduced processing speed. On the other hand, executive skills that involve reasoning about familiar material or appreciating the similarities between things seem to be well preserved with age.

It is perhaps useful to think of our intelligence – a measure of cognition – as either *crystallised* or *fluid*. Crystallised intelligence relates to abilities that have been well learnt and practised, such as general knowledge and vocabulary. Fluid intelligence, on the other hand, relates to our ability to 'think on the fly' and adapt to new situations, using skills that are less familiar and not directly associated with previous experiences. Examples of fluid intelligence include executive abilities, processing speed and memory function. Ageing affects fluid intelligence much more than crystallised intelligence. An individual who is ageing healthily keeps most of their base of underlying knowledge, though they may be slower to react to new and unfamiliar scenarios.

Natural versus pathological cognitive changes

In summary, there are some age-related cognitive changes that are potentially to be expected with healthy ageing:

- Slowed thinking
- More difficulty in finding the right word
- A deterioration in the ability to form new memories, and to recall the details of previous memories

- A reduction in executive abilities, especially those affected by speed of thinking.

Yet deficits in certain cognitive skills should be regarded as suspicious. For instance, age alone does not generally account for a significant deterioration in language ability, vocabulary or general verbal skills. Although there may be some mild degradation of *explicit memory* (consciously remembered information), *procedural memories* (those outside of a person's awareness, like riding a bike) generally remain intact with increasing age. Likewise, visuospatial skills are largely immune to significant change from age.

It is also important to note that although age causes some reduction in ability to acquire new memories, once they have been learnt, the ability to retain the memories should remain unaffected. Retrieving the memory may take a little more coaxing (and time), however.

These cognitive changes, by contrast, may suggest a problem:

- A deterioration in the ability to speak or write, including vocabulary
- A deterioration in procedural abilities, such as driving a car
- A deterioration in visuospatial abilities
- An inability to remember the broader aspects of things that have previously been well learnt.

Now that we have an understanding of how the brain's abilities may deteriorate with age, let's look at what we can do to minimise the impact of this, and hopefully to delay or even prevent the onset of dementia.

3

Preventing Cognitive Decline

- Strategies to protect your brain should be put in place as early as possible – ideally, decades before dementia traditionally develops.

- Managing stress, sleeping adequately and exercising regularly are important factors in maintaining brain health. Using your brain in challenging and novel ways is also critical.

- It is important to eat healthily. Following a Mediterranean diet or MIND diet seems to be especially protective against cognitive decline, and looking after your vascular health is vital.

- It is also helpful to socialise, optimise your hearing and be mindful of alcohol usage.

- Caloric restriction and fasting may help, but more research is needed and these interventions are not without risk.

The absence of a cure for dementia highlights the importance of trying to prevent or at least delay the condition, and research has revealed promising findings about what we can all do to protect ourselves. A recent study commissioned by *The Lancet*, a world-leading medical journal, estimated that about one third of dementia cases could be potentially eliminated if we as a population addressed a number of risk factors. Even if dementia cannot be prevented, pushing back its onset by a number of years – increasing our so-called healthspan – is a realistic and worthwhile goal.

I have developed an acronym – BRAINSCAN – that summarises the things we can all do to help preserve our brain function:

Be calm and happy
Restorative sleep
Active body
Investigate vascular health
Nurture friendships and socialise
Say what? Correct hearing loss
Complex mental activity
Alcohol awareness
Nourishing food

There is no hierarchy to the elements of BRAINSCAN. For each individual, though, some elements may have increased relevance: for instance, if there is a personal or family history of cardiovascular disease, heart health may be a particular focus. It is also important to recognise that the sooner these factors are addressed, the better. The damage that may eventually result in dementia can occur years or decades before the disease is apparent. Trying to address these concerns from midlife, if not earlier, is therefore very important.

Let's examine these elements of prevention and delay in more detail, starting with mental health.

Be calm and happy

Optimising our mental health is, for many, easier said than done. The two most common forms of mental unwellness – depression and anxiety – can both cause cognitive problems, and this is a good reason for us to look at our lives and ensure we are doing all we can to stay mentally healthy.

Common mental health conditions may cause an acute impairment in our cognitive ability while we are actively experiencing symptoms, but they may also cause chronic damage to the brain, mediated by (for instance) inflammatory processes and hormonal changes. We will discuss this in detail in Chapter 5, but for now it is important to note that there are effective treatments – from lifestyle and practical problem-solving interventions to more formal psychological therapies and, if need be, medications that can be very helpful in both the short and longer term.

Restorative sleep

When we sleep, new memories are replayed time and time again by the hippocampus, and distributed to other parts of the brain, where they become long-term memories available for future recall. Sleep therefore consolidates memory, and poor sleep interferes with this process. Also, sleep has been associated with the growth of new nerve cells in the brain, including in our hippocampus, a structure critical for memory formation.

One intriguing discovery a few years ago – of a network of specialised vessels in the brain known as the *glymphatic system* – has led to a biologically plausible theory linking sleeping problems with Alzheimer's disease and other chronic health conditions. The glymphatic system is thought to be a drainage system for clearing inflammatory molecules and beta-amyloid and tau proteins from the brain. These proteins are associated with Alzheimer's disease. The glymphatic system appears to be most active when we sleep (especially in the deepest stages), and studies have demonstrated that poor sleep leads to impaired clearance of amyloid and tau, increasing the risk of developing Alzheimer's disease. The amount of beta-amyloid in the brain increases after just one night of sleep deprivation, and chronically poor sleep has been associated with an increase in tau.

Poor sleep has also been associated with insulin resistance. The hormone insulin moves sugar (glucose) from the blood into the cells for energy. When we are resistant to its effects, there is more glucose circulating in our bloodstream, which raises the risk of type 2 diabetes, a condition associated with poor vascular health and cognitive impairment. Insulin resistance itself may also increase the deposition of beta-amyloid in the brain, increasing the risk of

Alzheimer's disease. Adding to this problem, disturbance of other hormones through poor sleep interferes with our appetite control, potentially leading to obesity – which, if chronic and developing in midlife particularly, may be another risk factor for dementia.

Sleep disturbance is a well-recognised symptom of dementia. Sleep is controlled by various structures in the brain, including the brainstem and the frontal areas, and the damage wrought to these by Alzheimer's disease or other causes of dementia may lead to numerous sleep difficulties. The evolving research dicussed above suggests, however, that the relationship is bidirectional.

It is important to recognise that although there seems to be a correlation between complaints of sleep disturbance earlier in life (specifically sleeping less than seven hours or over nine hours) and the later development of dementia, many people have chronic sleep problems but do not develop the condition. Nonetheless, the findings from studies on the issue do suggest that we should value and prioritise our sleep more than many of us do.

Both the quantity of sleep (seven to nine hours is ideal) and the quality is important. Even if you are sleeping for long enough, persistent fatigue or an inability to perform your usual daytime activities due to tiredness are causes for concern. Sleep can be impacted by numerous conditions both psychological and physical (notably sleep apnoea). If you are chronically sleep-deprived, it is worth discussing with your doctor.

There are also well-known lifestyle interventions that can help with sleep, collectively known as *sleep hygiene*. Examples include:

- Ensuring adequate daytime exposure to natural light
- Avoiding alcohol, caffeine and large meals later in the day
- Limiting daytime naps to less than 30 minutes
- Ensuring that you go to bed and get up at the same time each day (setting an alarm to go to bed is a helpful intervention for some)
- Establishing a regular and relaxing routine in the hours before bed
- Reducing lighting and screen-time in the evenings

- Engaging in regular physical exercise (but not late in the day, when the stimulating effect of exercise may prevent initiation of sleep)
- Ensuring that the bedtime environment is optimal: dark, quiet, physically comfortable and cool (about 16 degrees Celsius).

Active body

Humans are designed to be physically active; unfortunately for many of us, myself included, when we consistently fail to be so a multitude of health conditions may develop. These include vascular diseases (atherosclerosis, high cholesterol, high blood pressure, heart attacks and strokes), type 2 diabetes and some cancers (bowel, breast and cancer of the womb). When inactivity is combined with being overweight (which is of course more likely to occur because of inactivity), the risk of these problems occurring is even higher.

Cognitive impairment, including dementia, is also more likely to occur when someone is chronically physically inactive – it may account for as much as 14 per cent of the overall risk. Midlife obesity is also associated with a higher risk of dementia (though being overweight in later life is *not* a risk factor for cognitive decline and may in fact be protective). Nonetheless, this is encouraging news, as it means that we may be able to substantially reduce our chances of getting dementia by engaging in regular physical exercise and watching our weight, especially in our middle years.

It is likely that the earlier we attend to regular exercise in our lives, the more benefit it will give. Exercise has been robustly linked to improved executive function and processing speed in the cognitively healthy, and also in those with syndromes of cognitive impairment that are more than age-related but not as severe as dementia. These are known as *mild cognitive impairment* (MCI) and *subjective cognitive impairment* (SCI). (See Chapter 6 for a detailed discussion of these conditions.) Studies looking at exercise and memory function specifically have shown mixed results.

Some studies have demonstrated improved cognitive function for those who exercise even after dementia has set in. I encourage exercise in all my patients, regardless of their cognitive status. There are a host of other benefits of exercise, of course, including improved psychological wellbeing, improved sleep, maintenance of physical strength and a reduced risk of falls.

The most obvious way in which exercise can improve brain health is through its beneficial effect on our cardiovascular and cerebrovascular health. Exercising regularly is associated with better blood pressure control, improved cholesterol and blood sugar levels, and improved blood flow within our blood vessels. This translates to less vascular damage to the brain, and therefore less potential for cognitive impairment.

There are a number of other mechanisms by which exercise may confer cognitive benefit. In animals, it has been shown to increase the growth of nerve cells (*neurogenesis*) and the levels of chemicals that are thought to promote this growth (such as *brain-derived neurotrophic factor*). Inflammatory brain changes also seem to be ameliorated by exercise, and inflammation may play an important role in the genesis of dementia. Exercise also causes a reduction in brain beta-amyloid, the deposition of which is associated with Alzheimer's disease. Finally, it has been shown that exercise seems to help preserve the volume of certain brain structures, including the hippocampus, the structure responsible for new learning and which is an early target of Alzheimer's disease.

What sort of exercise is best? Well, it seems that a combination of aerobic activity (such as walking briskly, running, cycling or swimming) and strength training confers the greatest benefits. Aerobic exercise should ideally be strenuous enough to get you out of breath (you should be able to have a conversation but not sing!). The exact amount of exercise needed remains unclear, though 150 minutes of moderate exercise per week is a general health guideline and one that is worth striving for. Walking briskly for 30 minutes, five times a week, is a common recommendation.

It also makes intuitive sense to regularly change the sort of exercise to get the most benefit – perhaps walking twice a week, swimming a couple of times, and doing some resistance (or weight) training on the other days. There is some evidence that this latter form of exercise may be particularly beneficial if it is progressive or graduated – that is, the heaviness of the weights is increased from session to session.

One additional interesting finding is that when exercise has a social aspect – that is, when it's done in a group setting – the cognitive benefits appear to be greater than when it's done alone. Why this should be so is not entirely clear, though socialisation itself is a cognitive task and this may be relevant.

Ageing may cause physical impediments to exercise, such as pain, muscle weakness and cardiac or respiratory disease, but these hurdles can often be overcome by being flexible and creative. A physiotherapist or exercise physiologist can advise on how to create a personalised exercise plan that is safe and practical.

Investigate vascular health

Vascular disease refers to disease affecting the blood supply to various parts of the body. It includes cerebrovascular (to the brain) and cardiovascular (to the heart) disease.

Vascular disease is indisputably a risk factor for dementia, and not only vascular dementia. A 2009 study, which had followed individuals over 30 years, reported that those with high cholesterol in midlife had higher rates of dementia in later life; a more recent study demonstrated a clearer causal link, showing that those with at least two risk factors for vascular disease in midlife had a higher rate of beta-amyloid in their brain (as measured using scans) in later life. This study also showed that the more risk factors were present, the more beta-amyloid was present. Having vascular disease therefore seems to increase the risk of developing Alzheimer's disease.

Vascular risk factors include obesity, high cholesterol, diabetes, a sedentary lifestyle, a family history of vascular disease, and smoking. Most of these are amenable to treatment, and addressing them can be of great benefit in reducing the risk of dementia. Ideally, the efforts to do so should happen in midlife, many years before the condition usually presents.

The MIND diet, which attempts to address one of the vascular risk factors, high blood pressure, has been shown to be of benefit in reducing the impact of this risk factor. We'll explore this in more detail later in this chapter, but I strongly recommend that you discuss assessment and treatment of vascular disease with your GP. Vascular dementia itself is covered in Chapter 8.

Nurture friendships and socialise

Just as we are designed to move, so too are we designed to socialise. This desire to connect and share experiences with others is an innately human quality, having conferred joy as well as a survival advantage since the early days of human evolution.

It is worth noting the distinction between *social isolation* and *loneliness*, as they are not the same thing. Social isolation is a *situation* in which a person has limited contact with other people. Loneliness is a negative *feeling* that may or may not occur when social isolation is present. Some individuals may have very limited social contact but not feel lonely, and others may be surrounded by people – in an aged-care facility, for example – but still feel alone. When we look at risk factors for dementia, it is the feeling of loneliness rather than the degree of social contact that is most important.

Social contact and a sense of connection to others is highly protective in a number of ways, and its absence is associated with a host of adverse health outcomes. These include physical conditions, such as cardiovascular disease, breast cancer and infectious diseases, and psychological ones, including depression and anxiety. Some of these conditions themselves increase the risk of dementia and add to the direct impact of loneliness upon dementia risk.

Although we may not recognise it as so, socialising – the process of engaging with, and actively listening to and responding to other people – is a cognitive task and exercises the brain. This may be one of the reasons that socialising is protective. As with exercise, there may be additional benefits from engaging in different activities – socialising with family and with different groups of friends.

Say what? Correct hearing loss

Hearing loss has also been associated with Alzheimer's disease, with a doubling of the risk of developing the latter condition if the hearing loss is mild, and up to a fivefold risk when it is severe. These findings were obtained by examining individuals with hearing loss in midlife (defined as 45–65 years of age) and determining their rate of dementia over the following ten years or so. This raises the importance of having one's hearing loss treated many years before dementia traditionally occurs.

The mechanism by which hearing loss may increase the risk of dementia remains unclear. It may increase social isolation and feelings of loneliness or depression, or may require the brain to allocate more resources to hearing and decoding words at the expense of memory function and other cognitive tasks. It is feasible also that the same process causing the dementia is also responsible for the hearing loss.

Regardless of the mechanism, it has been estimated that correcting hearing loss in midlife could reduce the number of new cases of later dementia by 9 per cent, which is considerably more than other midlife factors. (The same study considered that addressing high blood pressure could reduce the risk by 2 per cent, and addressing obesity by 1 per cent.) Some studies have been conducted (others are in progress) to establish whether the use of devices to improve hearing, such as hearing aids and cochlear implants, can prevent or slow the onset of dementia. The evidence so far is encouraging. One study on cochlear implants demonstrated that the cognitive benefits of using such a device were twice as impressive as those achieved by using cholinesterase inhibitors – one of only two types of medication we have at our disposal to improve cognition in those with dementia.

Symptoms of mild hearing loss include perceiving a muffling of speech and other sounds, having difficulty understanding words (especially when there is background noise), having trouble hearing consonants in particular, needing to turn up the TV or radio, and withdrawing from social contact owing to an inability to hear well. Discuss any symptoms of hearing loss with your GP; they can be formally assessed by an audiologist.

Complex mental activity

Underpinning the discussion about mental activity and cognitive performance is the concept of *neurogenesis*. This term describes the creation of nerve cells from stem cells, the basic cells that populate our body before they become specialised. Although it is not without controversy, the prevailing view is that neurogenesis continues throughout life, including in areas of the brain responsible for learning. An associated term is *neuroplasticity*, which highlights that things we do are able to change the architecture of our brain networks in a helpful fashion.

One of the other terms often used in discussions surrounding dementia is *cognitive reserve*. This refers to the ability of the brain to maintain its function despite being damaged by, for instance, vascular disease or beta-amyloid protein. Brains with good cognitive reserve have a robust capacity to compensate for these disease processes, perhaps by using other brain areas or processes. This compensation allows an individual to maintain a higher degree of day-to-day function.

Cognitive reserve is affected by a number of things, including unmodifiable factors such as our genetics and age, but also factors we have control over, such as socialising and the amount of *complex mental activity* we engage in. This mental activity influences dementia risk from childhood, when our brains are rapidly developing, and continues to affect the risk well into our middle adulthood. It does so by promoting neurogenesis.

But what do we mean by complex mental activity? Well, despite its name, it is a relatively simple concept, if somewhat ill-defined. Complex mental activity really refers to mentally stimulating or taxing activities – ones that make you think hard and force you to purposefully engage in the task at hand. Examples include completing a crossword or sudoku, learning a new hobby, performing tai chi, taking up sailing, learning to dance, trying to master a new language, cooking an unfamiliar recipe, or undertaking formal study.

Higher educational levels have been associated with a reduction in the risk of dementia, and it is likely that occupations which are more cognitively challenging confer some benefit by increasing cognitive reserve. A high degree of social engagement over the years may also be protective against memory loss later in life.

Other factors are likely to influence the impact of complex mental activity on delaying dementia. One is novelty – that is, it is probably more beneficial to engage in tasks in which we are naturally less skilled or practised. Perennial crossword addicts would be better off tackling a sudoku, and vice versa. Learning in a group setting may also provide greater cognitive benefit than learning alone.

Given the above, it seems reasonable to surmise that if we exercise our brain in a formal and standardised way, this will help increase our cognitive reserve and stave off later cognitive problems. This is the theoretical benefit of the many 'brain training' programs that exist (such as Lumosity, Elevate, HappyNeuron, BrainHQ, CogniFit and MyBrainTrainer). These programs usually include a number of visually appealing and engaging games that are designed to exercise different aspects of cognition – whether that be visual memory, processing speed, visuospatial abilities or something else.

Do these interventions help? Unfortunately that remains unclear. Many studies have demonstrated improvements in the specific areas of cognitive function being exercised. What is less certain is whether this translates to meaningful changes in everyday function. Generalisability is the key issue. One study – the ACTIVE study, which involved assessing almost 3000 individuals – did show a translated everyday improvement, though the authors noted that it took many years to become evident. Interestingly, a study by the Queensland Brain Institute showed that stimulating the prefrontal cortex with an electrical charge seemed to help cement improvement in performance *as well as* helping performance on other cognitive tasks. This is a promising area of research.

No harm has been associated with formal cognitive training, and if individuals are not restricted financially and are keen on using such programs, I do not dissuade them – as long it is not causing them stress. If it is, then often the whole process is counterproductive, with stress itself known to impair cognitive function.

Alcohol awareness

Chronic excessive use of alcohol is likely to increase the risk of developing dementia. Alcohol is, after all, a neurotoxin, and the brain only has a limited ability to absorb its impact. The relationship between lower levels of alcohol consumption and dementia is more complicated, however. Chapter 9 includes a dedicated discussion on this topic.

Nourishing food

One of the most encouraging areas of research into preventing or delaying cognitive decline and dementia concerns diet. Healthy dietary choices can substantially reduce the risk of developing these conditions, especially if begun early in life.

The following aspects of diet have been associated with a lower risk of developing dementia.

Lower intake of saturated and trans-unsaturated fats

These are the 'bad' fats, typically found in junk food and fast food. Dairy products contain saturated fats, as do certain fatty meats. Coconut oil and full-fat milk are high in saturated fat. Many cakes, pastries, pies and deep-fried foods contain both saturated and trans fats. The damage these compounds cause is not restricted to dementia – they can cause problems in all areas of our physical (and probably mental) health. A small amount of saturated fat in one's diet is unlikely to be deleterious if you are otherwise healthy. There is no room for trans fats in a healthy diet, however.

Higher intake of omega 3 fats

These are found in oily fish such as salmon, tuna and sardines, which it is recommended we eat two to three times a week. They are also found in certain nuts and seeds, especially flaxseed and walnuts, and can be taken in the form of supplements. The evidence suggests, however, that when dementia 'sets in', increasing the intake of omega 3 fats may not be helpful.

Higher intake of monounsaturated and polyunsaturated fats
These are the 'good' fats and are found in numerous foods, including olives (and olive oil), certain other oils (canola, sunflower), nuts and avocados.

Higher intake of vegetables and fruit
Many of these contain valuable antioxidants, helpful for addressing chronic inflammation. More deeply or brightly coloured fruits and vegetables contain greater quantities of antioxidants.

Adequate intake of B group vitamins
Low levels of vitamin B9 (folate) and vitamin B12 in particular may be associated with an increased risk of dementia. B12 can be found in meat, shellfish, dairy foods, tempeh and some fortified breakfast cereals. Sources of folate include leafy vegetables such as spinach, legumes (chickpeas, lentils, peas and peanuts) and certain fruits and vegetables, including avocados, oranges, bananas, rockmelon and strawberries. B vitamins also come in the form of supplements.

Improving your dietary choices

Much of the increased risk of dementia due to certain dietary choices seems to be related to the impact of poor diet on heart disease (including high blood pressure and high cholesterol) and stroke. High cholesterol may increase the production of beta-amyloid. Excessive sugar intake may also cause or worsen diabetes, which also increases the risk of dementia.

Some studies have demonstrated that, even without formally causing diabetes, chronic high sugar intake can hasten cognitive decline, perhaps through promoting insulin resistance and inflammatory changes. In addition, obesity and high-fat diets have been shown to increase inflammation in the brain, which can damage cells and impair brain function.

Diets for health and weight loss go in and out of fashion. It is hard to judge their merits from a cognitive perspective – unfortunately, for the majority, including currently fashionable options such as the ketogenic and paleo diets, we do not have good evidence to either support or dismiss their use. An additional concern is that some of these diets may lead to unhealthy weight loss or deprive individuals of vital nutrients. This is especially relevant in the elderly and if used long term.

The two dietary strategies that do have reasonably robust data to recommend them for cognition are the Mediterranean diet and the MIND diet.

The Mediterranean diet

This dietary approach has been shown to be protective for heart and brain health, and those using this diet have a lower risk of developing dementia (as well as other chronic diseases). The main components of this diet are:

- Eating primarily plant-based foods, such as fruits and vegetables, whole grains, legumes and nuts
- Using herbs and spices (instead of salt) to flavour food
- Eating fish and poultry at least twice a week
- Limiting red meat to no more than a few times a month
- Drinking red wine in moderation (optional!)
- Replacing butter with healthy fats such as olive oil and canola.

There are other indirect elements of the Mediterranean diet that may be protective against dementia, including the social aspect (eating with family and friends) and getting regular physical exercise.

The MIND diet

This eating approach combines the Mediterranean diet with the Dietary Approaches to Stop Hypertension diet, producing the Mediterranean-DASH Intervention for Neurodegenerative Delay diet, or MIND diet. It has also shown evidence of benefit, with those most rigorously following it being the equivalent of 7.5 years younger cognitively than those least following it. This cognitive advantage has been shown to be even stronger in elderly individuals who have suffered a stroke.

The MIND diet includes the following:

- Six or more servings of green leafy vegetables (kale, spinach, cooked greens, salads) per week
- One or more additional serve of another vegetable per day – preferably a non-starchy one
- Five or more servings of nuts per week (the type of nut is not specified, though eating a variety makes nutritional sense)
- Two servings of berries (strawberries, blueberries, raspberries or blackberries) per week
- Three serves of whole grains per day (options include brown rice, whole wheat pasta, 100 per cent whole wheat bread, quinoa)
- Four servings of beans per week
- Olive oil as the main cooking oil
- One serve of fish per week (it is preferable to eat fatty fish such as salmon, trout, sardines or mackerel, as these contain high levels of omega 3 fatty acids)
- Two serves of chicken or turkey per week
- No more than one glass of wine per day
- Less than one tablespoon of butter or margarine per day
- Less than one serving of cheese per week
- No more than three servings of red meat per week
- Minimal fried food, pastries and sweets.

It is important to note that this advice is based on evidence about reducing the risk of dementia developing in the first place. Research looking at changing the course of dementia once it is present is currently lacking. It is intuitive, however, that the same advice should apply (perhaps aside from drinking alcohol), regardless of whether dementia has set in or not.

In summary, diet is a critical element of reducing the risk of cognitive impairment and dementia, and good dietary choices in the years and even decades before dementia classically develops can be highly protective. Using the Mediterranean or MIND diet appears to have the most robust evidence, though avoidance of chronic excessive sugar intake – not especially mentioned in these diets – also appears wise, as does regular intake of foods with antioxidant properties.

Fasting – an honourable mention

Caloric restriction – the limiting of calories consumed through food – is one of the few interventions that has been shown to increase lifespan, at least in animal studies. It has been shown to have beneficial effects on a number of chronic health conditions, including diabetes, obesity, certain cancers and cardiovascular disease. One way of achieving caloric restriction is through *intermittent fasting*, and research has been undertaken to see if this may help stave off cognitive decline, including dementia. The idea has merit, as we know that fasting creates a state conducive to reducing inflammation, and chronic inflammation may play a role in cognitive decline.

So, what does the research tell us? Well, that more research needs to be done! So far, most studies have been done on animals, though a few have been done on healthy older adults and those with mild cognitive impairment. These studies have generally yielded positive results, with improved cognition noted in those who fasted, but further study is required. It should also be noted that prolonged fasting is not without its own risks, particularly in the frail and elderly.

Next we'll look at the role of supplements and minerals in preventing cognitive decline.

4

Supplements and Vitamins in Cognition

- Many supplements are thought to work through their antioxidant and anti-inflammatory actions.

- A number of small studies have indicated that supplements may be helpful in maintaining a healthy brain, but we do not have robust evidence to support supplement use in someone who is otherwise healthy. They are more likely to be beneficial in those with a deficiency.

- Likewise, we cannot say conclusively whether supplements will be of help to someone with dementia. More research is required.

- A supplement may be 'natural' but that does not mean taking it is without risk. Any chemical we put in our body has the potential to cause problems, or may interact with prescribed medications.

- Naturally occurring compounds are probably more effective when taken as part of our diet rather than in supplement form.

- The evidence regarding the impact of hormone replacement therapy on cognitive function is not conclusive.

A large number of supplements, vitamins and minerals claim to offer protection against dementia; every week seems to bring another article extolling the virtues of a new miracle product. I am frequently asked about such supplements in my clinic. Some are 'old familiars', having been in the public eye for some time, but many have been unfamiliar to me. Often these latter substances ride a wave of clever marketing and social media, and are not based on good evidence.

One particularly concerning aspect of many supplements is that they have not been tested with the rigour that is applied to prescribed medications, and so their safety profile is unclear. Such supplements may also interact problematically with other medications an individual may be taking.

An exhaustive list of every product spruiked for cognitive enhancement would be a book in itself. Below, however, I have highlighted the more commonly discussed supplements, some of which may be very familiar.

Souvenaid

Souvenaid is a milky drink developed specifically to optimise brain nutrition. It contains a combination of fatty acids, vitamins and other nutrients, and has been around for over ten years. Studies of its effectiveness have shown mixed results, making it difficult to be conclusive about whether it helps with dementia. Tests performed on animals have shown promising results, but tests on humans have been less compelling.

A relatively large study published in 2017 – in which individuals with prodromal Alzheimer's disease (that is, where there was evidence from brain scans or lumbar punctures of Alzheimer's disease, but insufficient clinical signs to warrant a diagnosis) were assigned either to a group taking Souvenaid or to a group not taking it. The study found no significant change overall in cognitive functioning, although those using the drink did seem to fare better when their dementia was rated according to functional impact (using the Clinical Dementia Rating scale). They also demonstrated slowed shrinkage of the hippocampus, critical for memory retention. The results were considered encouraging but not conclusive.

Souvenaid may be of some benefit where Alzheimer's disease is mild, though it is not considered appropriate for those in the moderate to severe stages of the illness. There is insufficient information on its use in those with other dementias or MCI.

Souvenaid comes in small bottles available to buy from pharmacies, and one bottle is drunk per day. They cost about the same as a cup of coffee. It is well tolerated: only mild side effects (diarrhoea, dizziness and headache) have been reported. It may not be suitable for those with allergies to fish/seafood, soy or milk, however.

A number of patients have come to me on a combination of various nutrients and supplements, many of which have not been studied at all in relation to dementia. If they appear to have mild Alzheimer's disease, I often suggest they take Souvenaid as a convenient alternative to these other, often costly products, many of which may have unpredictable side effects. We at least know that Souvenaid is safe and it *may* help, although clearly more research needs to be done.

Ginkgo biloba

This herbal supplement, used in Chinese medicine for centuries, has been studied in relation to dementia, though the studies are considered to be of low quality, which limits what advice can be given about its use. It is thought to work through improving blood circulation and may also have antioxidant effects, though its precise mechanism of action remains unclear.

An overview of systematic reviews published in 2017 noted the low quality of evidence, but concluded there may be some benefit for those with dementia when it is used consistently for five months or more at a dose of 200 milligrams per day.

Studies have also compared treatment with ginkgo biloba versus treatment with cholinesterase inhibitors. These latter medications are used to treat the cognitive problems associated with some types of dementia, particularly dementia due to Alzheimer's disease. The results of these studies have varied. Some suggest it to be as effective as cholinesterase inhibitors and some show it to be less effective. It is also unclear whether there is any added benefit when the two types of medication are combined.

One of the benefits of ginkgo biloba is that it is well tolerated. Minor side effects include stomach upset, dizziness, constipation and headaches. It can, however, interact with medications designed to thin the blood (such as warfarin and aspirin) and those that inadvertently do so (such as ibuprofen and other anti-inflammatories), and I would tend to advise against its use in people taking these medications or who are at higher risk of internal bleeding.

More research is required to establish the role of ginkgo biloba in preventing and treating dementia.

Brahmi

Also known as bacopa, brahmi is a plant that is used in Ayurvedic medicine. It is considered to have antioxidant and anti-inflammatory effects and may increase dilation of blood vessels, thereby improving brain blood flow. All these mechanisms could theoretically be helpful in reducing the impact of dementia. In animals, brahmi has also been shown to have an anti-amyloid effect.

One study from 2002 demonstrated a protective effect of brahmi in individuals *without* dementia against forgetting newly acquired information, though it failed to identify improvements in other cognitive skills. The improvement in forgetting is consistent with an observed antioxidant effect of brahmi on the hippocampus in rats, which could mean less oxidative stress-related damage to these structures. (See Chapter 8 for a discussion of oxidative stress.)

Brahmi's solitary positive effect on 'memory free recall' has been backed up by some other studies, but not all. A review of the evidence in 2013 concluded that there is some evidence to support the idea that brahmi improves this area of thinking, but not enough evidence to comment greatly on other areas of cognition – in part because of inconsistent measures of cognition used across the different studies. It seems, then, that more research is needed to make confident judgements about its effect, even in people with no clinical diagnosis of dementia.

A more recent review on the use of brahmi concluded that although a number of animal studies suggested it may be a promising treatment, there are insufficient studies in humans to assess its effectiveness and safety in those experiencing dementia. More research is needed.

On the whole, brahmi appears to be tolerated well, although it can cause stomach cramps, diarrhoea, nausea and fatigue. Its long-term effects, however, have not been extensively researched.

Vitamin E

Vitamin E is thought to have an antioxidant effect, a property that could theoretically make it helpful in treating cognitive impairment, including dementia, although there is insufficient evidence to conclude that it is effective. There are also concerns that vitamin E, when taken as a supplement, may increase the risk of internal bleeding. Anyone on blood-thinning agents such as aspirin, warfarin or clopidogrel should be especially aware of this issue.

Omega 3 fatty acids

Found in oily fish (salmon, tuna and sardines) and certain nuts and seeds (walnuts and flaxseed especially), these compounds are considered to have a number of beneficial health effects mediated by their anti-inflammatory and antioxidant properties. They are available in capsule form from pharmacies.

Omega 3 fatty acids have been recommended for a number of chronic health conditions, including cardiovascular disease and arthritis. There is evidence that diets high in omega 3 fatty acids slow the rate of memory decline in people who do not have dementia but are at higher risk due to having an APOE4 allele. (For discussion of this risk factor, see Chapter 8.) On the other hand, studies looking more generally at cognitively healthy individuals who are not in this higher risk category have failed to demonstrate any benefit from taking omega 3 as a supplement. A number of good-quality studies have also failed to demonstrate any benefit in people who already have mild to moderate Alzheimer's disease.

When taken in the recommended dose, omega 3 fatty acid supplements are unlikely to do any harm, though they can promote bleeding and so should be used with caution by those with bleeding tendencies or those on other medications that may thin the blood (anti-inflammatories, aspirin, warfarin and so on). The side effects are generally mild; they include halitosis (bad breath), nausea and diarrhoea, and heartburn.

It would seem preferable, given the evidence we have, to try to consume omega 3 fatty acids as part our diet rather than in pill form. Oily fish is a more potent source than plants and represents one of the ingredients of the Mediterranean diet (discussed in Chapter 3), which is thought to be neuroprotective.

Curcumin

This naturally occurring molecule is found in the root of turmeric, a spice native to the Indian subcontinent. Interest in this compound has been spearheaded by the finding that in India, where it is a common component of curry, there is a low incidence of Alzheimer's disease. It is thought to have antioxidant, anti-inflammatory and, in particular, anti-amyloid effects.

One of the difficulties in researching this molecule in relation to Alzheimer's disease is the unpredictability of its absorption into the body and of how much of it may get to the necessary sites of action (that is, the brain). Pharmaceutical companies are working to find formulations that are optimised in this regard. The optimal dose of curcumin also remains unclear.

A recent small study demonstrated that curcumin can help improve memory and attention in adults without dementia. Larger studies are required before a more conclusive understanding can be reached. Unfortunately, there is insufficient evidence to promote the use of curcumin in treating dementia at this stage.

Aspirin and anti-inflammatory medications

Due to their anti-inflammatory effect, aspirin and certain other analgesic medications (including naproxen, ibuprofen, diclofenac and celecoxib) could theoretically have a protective effect against Alzheimer's disease. Some early studies suggested that those taking non-steroidal anti-inflammatory drugs (known as NSAIDs) may have a reduced incidence of the disease. Subsequent clinical studies failed to show any benefit, however.

This style of medication can cause problems with internal bleeding and, for the NSAIDs, a number of other health problems, especially cardiac and renal conditions. For these reasons I do not recommend the use of these agents for the purposes of treating dementia (though they may still be appropriate for other purposes, of course).

Caffeine

Caffeine is one of the world's most widely used supplements, so much so that we do not really see it as such. For many of us it is part of daily life, contained in varying quantities in coffee, tea, caffeinated soft and alcoholic drinks, and chocolate.

Over the years, coffee consumption in particular has been associated with numerous health benefits, such as increased life span and reduced risk of numerous diseases, including Parkinson's disease, cardiovascular disease, type 2 diabetes, uterine and liver cancer, and cirrhosis. It may also be protective against depression. Although the reasons for these benefits are not entirely known, the caffeine component may well play a role. (The research often does not differentiate between caffeinated and decaffeinated coffee, however, which complicates interpretation of the results.)

It should also be noted that caffeine, for some, can cause adverse effects, including inducing anxiety and increasing pulse rate and modestly increasing blood pressure. There is a lot of individual variation when it comes to how well tolerated caffeine is, and there is certainly a relationship between the dose and the potential for side effects. Studies have previously demonstrated a possible link between caffeine and certain cancers, such as bladder and pancreatic cancer, though the findings have since been refuted. A link between oesophageal (throat) cancer and coffee has been largely attributed to the heat of the drink rather than to the caffeine contained within.

But what about caffeine's effect on cognition and dementia risk? Unfortunately, this remains an unanswered question. One of the mechanisms of the action of caffeine is through *adenosine receptors*. Adenosine is a neurotransmitter that, when bound to its receptor on a nerve cell, causes a reduction in activity that results in sleepiness and other changes such as dilation of blood vessels. Caffeine binds to these same receptors, meaning that adenosine cannot bind, and in this way it prevents the usual 'braking' effect of adenosine on the nervous system. This leads to improved alertness, and this in turn can improve cognitive performance while under the influence of the drug. In addition to alertness, attention and concentration have been shown consistently to improve with caffeine on board, and some studies have demonstrated benefits for memory and executive function.

Adenosine exerts some of its effects by reducing the release of various other neurotransmitters, including acetylcholine, glutamate and dopamine. These substances are critical for optimal brain function. By effectively reducing the activity of adenosine, caffeine indirectly increases the activity of these other substances, perhaps explaining the observed cognitive benefits noted above. Studies in mice have also shown that caffeine reduces beta-amyloid (associated with Alzheimer's disease) in the blood and brain.

The effect of caffeine on dementia risk has been studied on numerous occasions, though methodological issues have meant that we cannot draw strong conclusions. Nonetheless, an interesting study in 2012 showed that higher levels of caffeine in the blood were associated with a lower risk of developing dementia in those known to have MCI (see Chapter 6). Another study, the CAIDE study, demonstrated a link between midlife coffee consumption (of three to five cups per day) and a reduced rate of dementia later in life. A more recent study, conducted only on women, found an association between caffeine consumption in later life (in this study, between the ages of 65 and 80) and a reduced risk of dementia, though the effects are considered modest, and there has been criticism of how this study was conducted.

Although the use of caffeine may confer a number of benefits from a cognitive perspective and may exert a protective effect against progressive cognitive impairment and dementia, caution is advised in its use once the condition is manifest. The evidence, at least in studies of mice with Alzheimer's disease, suggests that consumption of caffeine is associated with an increase in behavioural and psychological symptoms.

I certainly do not dissuade moderate coffee drinkers from continuing their habit, as long as it is not causing any adverse effects, but individuals should be mindful of the limitations of the conclusions of research into caffeine and dementia.

B vitamins

As mentioned in the previous chapter, a link between a deficiency of certain B vitamins, especially cobalamin (B12), folate/folic acid (B9) and thiamine (B1), and cognitive impairment has been clearly established. Low levels of B12 in the blood has also been associated with increased brain atrophy, and therefore with increased risk of cognitive impairment. Treatment of these deficiencies can result in improvement of cognitive function.

The role of vitamin B supplements in those who are not deficient is a little less clear, however. A 2018 review that incorporated more than 27,000 people from various studies concluded that there was no advantage to B vitamin supplementation for those over 40 years of age who are cognitively healthy. There is little data on the routine use of B vitamin supplements for those who are not deficient but have MCI or dementia. Individuals with high blood homocysteine levels (a risk factor for Alzheimer's disease and vascular disease) may gain specific benefit, however. See Chapter 3 for an outline of good dietary sources of vitamin B.

Vitamin D

There is evidence that a severe deficiency of vitamin D (known as the 'sunshine vitamin', as this is our best source of it) may increase the risk of dementia. A recent study at the Queensland Brain Institute showed that vitamin D deficiency is associated with poorer performance on cognitive tests as well as with a reduced size of the hippocampus, often the first structure affected by Alzheimer's disease. The results of a 2014 study suggested that those with severely low vitamin D levels were twice as likely to develop dementia than those with adequate levels. Whether vitamin D is of any benefit in preventing or treating dementia when there is no deficiency has not been adequately studied, however.

Vitamin D levels are easily tested using a blood test, and any deficiency should be treated. Eggs, liver and fatty fish contain vitamin D, though the contribution of our diet to vitamin D levels is quite low. Vitamin D tablets can also be used, though this should be discussed with your GP. It should also be noted that excessive vitamin D – almost invariably the result of supplementation with tablets – can be harmful, causing kidney problems and bone pain.

Coconut oil

Among the purported health benefits of coconut oil is that it may help with brain health and cognition. It is almost 100 per cent fat, much of which is saturated, though the structure of this fat differs from that of many animal sources in that it mainly consists of medium-chain triglycerides (MCTs) rather than long-chain triglycerides (LCTs). Some researchers have shown that MCTs increase high-density lipoproteins (HDL – our 'good' cholesterol). Others have shown the opposite: that HDL cholesterol is reduced, leading to an increase in low-density lipoproteins (LDL – our 'bad' cholesterol) and therefore vascular disease.

Another potential cognitive benefit comes from the ability of coconut oil to provide a ready energy source (ketones) for the brain. Some believe that the brain cells of those with dementia may not be able to use glucose – their usual source of energy – well, perhaps related to problems with insulin resistance. Insulin helps direct glucose into cells, and with insulin resistance this ability is hampered. Coconut oil may therefore be a helpful alternative source. This theory has not really been rigorously tested, however.

In a story that is now familiar, the jury is out when it comes to coconut oil, cognitive performance and dementia. More research is needed to clarify the issue.

In summary

The take-home message in regard to these supplements and vitamins is that their role in optimising cognition and in preventing and treating dementia remains unclear, though some show promise. Studies that have attempted to assess their effectiveness have often been poorly conducted and show inconsistent results. We cannot say that they will help, but at the same time we cannot say that they won't. In situations where an individual is deficient in a particular vitamin, the argument for using a supplement is considerably stronger.

It is also important to note that these supplements may have side effects and cause problematic interactions with other medications. Hopefully there will be more robust investigation into these compounds, and others, in the future, which may allow us to draw more confident conclusions.

A note on HRT

Although hormone replacement therapy (HRT) does not really fit under the rubric of supplements, it is worth mentioning here. HRT involves the use of hormones (oestrogen and progesterone) whose levels in the body drop with the onset of menopause. Oestrogen, in particular, is thought to reduce the amount of beta-amyloid in the brain by mopping up free radicals and reducing oxidative stress.

There has been considerable controversy about the risks and benefits of HRT, not only in relation to cognition. The evidence suggests that the risk of breast cancer, endometrial cancer (cancer of the womb) and ovarian cancer is increased by certain formulations (oestrogen-only formulations), and so even if there were a benefit cognitively in having HRT, these risks would need to be considered.

Studies looking at HRT as a preventive against dementia have shown mixed results. Some have demonstrated a small benefit, others no benefit, and some the opposite – that taking HRT may in fact increase the risk of Alzheimer's disease if it is taken in the long term (over a number of years) as a pill. This is a tricky area, and one which needs further research before conclusive advice can be given. At the current time, however, HRT is not recommended for treating cognitive symptoms associated with perimenopause and menopause.

In the next part of the book, we will examine the various causes of cognitive impairment in more detail.

SECTION II
Defining Dementia

5

Reversible Cognitive Impairment

- It is important to be alert for reversible causes of cognitive impairment. They may be the sole cause of the problem or complicate the cognitive problems in dementia.

- Depression, anxiety and other psychological conditions can impair our thinking. If they are long-term problems, they may increase the risk of dementia. Sometimes, however, these psychological disturbances can be an early sign of dementia.

- A variety of physical health conditions can cause cognitive impairment and may also exacerbate the cognitive symptoms of dementia. These need to be ruled out.

- Perimenopause is a natural phenomenon that can cause cognitive impairment, but it resolves and its occurrence does not indicate a greater risk of dementia.

- Multiple medications, alone or especially in combination, can also cause symptoms that look like dementia.

- Delirium is a very common cause of confusion and can be mistaken for dementia, though it has a distinctive profile that helps differentiate it.

Everyone who comes to see me about their cognitive problems hopes we will discover a cause that, when treated, will result in complete resolution of their symptoms. Although this does not eventuate in the majority of the cases I see (and studies show highly varying rates of reversible causes of apparent dementia), sometimes it does happen and it is crucial that these are recognised. Dementia, by contrast, is permanent and progressive.

Reversible causes of cognitive impairment can be grouped into three categories: psychological conditions, physical causes and those caused by prescribed or non-prescribed drugs. We will address each in turn.

Psychological conditions that may cause cognitive impairment

In my work as a psychiatrist with both the elderly and younger adults, I see patients who have a variety of troubling psychological illnesses. These include depression, anxiety disorders and conditions where there are psychotic symptoms, such as delusions and hallucinations. Some of these can cause cognitive problems that are reversible.

Depression

Perhaps the most important psychological condition that may cause problems with cognition is depression. Along with anxiety, it is one of the most common mental health disorders in the world.

It is unusual for depression in earlier life to cause memory and other cognitive deficits severe enough to be misinterpreted as dementia. In later years, though, the situation is different. This may have something to do with reduced cognitive reserve. That is, the brain is more vulnerable, through the effects of ageing and other comorbid problems, to the cogni-toxic impact of depression. When cognitive impairment resembles dementia but is actually caused by depression, it is known as *depressive pseudodementia*.

One important issue here is the overlap and interface between dementia and depression. The risk of depression is greater in those with dementia. Depression can also be the first manifestation of the condition. Depressive episodes may occur a number of years before the more recognisable cognitive symptoms of dementia develop. In one large study, individuals who had experienced anxiety and depression symptoms in middle age were 20 per cent more likely to develop dementia later in life.

The possibility that episodes of depression earlier in life may be a risk factor for later dementia has also been examined: a few studies seem to indicate that it is and have shown a correlation between dementia risk and the severity of depression as well as the number of episodes – a so-called 'dose effect'. Other studies have not shown a relationship. The debate therefore is unresolved. In one study, at least, it has been shown that major depression and chronic stress may cause loss of brain volume contributing to mild cognitive impairment (MCI), which is associated with an increased risk of dementia. Depression is also associated with high cortisol levels, and chronically high levels of this 'stress hormone' have been associated with cognitive decline. Furthermore, depression has been associated specifically with reduced hippocampal size, a cardinal early feature of Alzheimer's disease.

How do we assess whether someone is depressed? Well, a diagnosis of depression is based primarily on the presence of other, non-cognitive symptoms, and we therefore ask about these:

- Consistently low mood
- A lack of energy
- A lack of interest and pleasure
- Reduced sex drive
- Indecisiveness
- A slowing of thought and movement noticeable to others
- Disturbance of sleep and/or appetite
- Feelings of hopelessness or helplessness
- A belief that one would be better off dead, or suicidal thinking.

In the elderly, anxiety and agitation can be especially prominent features of a depressive syndrome, and somatic symptoms (unexplained physical symptoms like general aches and pains) are not uncommon. In severe cases, there may be psychotic features (false beliefs or hallucinations). These are typically *mood-congruent*; that is, the themes of the delusions mirror the mood state. Examples are delusions of poverty, delusions of guilt, or delusional beliefs that one has a terrible illness such as cancer, or that one should be punished.

Some of these symptoms may also occur as part of a dementia itself – for example, loss of interest, slowing of thought, or sleep disturbance – and it is important to establish whether dementia or depression is the primary driver.

The cognitive difficulties associated with depression differ in significant ways from those seen in dementia alone. One important factor is the impact of poor motivation and low self-confidence. This results in individuals performing poorly on cognitive testing simply because they lack the motivation to complete the tasks. They may respond to memory questions by saying, 'I don't know,' but when they are encouraged, they are often able to complete the task. Areas of cognition impacted particularly by depression include processing speed, attention, executive function, learning and memory.

With my elderly patients, I often use the Geriatric Depression Scale. This is a well-validated screening tool that can be viewed online. It assumes that the person being assessed does not have a significant dementia.

If there is evidence of a depressive illness, it is important to treat this before coming to any definitive conclusion about the presence or severity of an underlying dementia. The latter condition may well still exist, though even if it does, depression can make it seem much worse than it is.

The following table sets out some of the features that can help distinguish between dementia and depressive pseudodementia.

Clinical feature	Depressive pseudodementia	Dementia
Onset	Over weeks to months	Over years (usually)
Pattern of low mood	Persistently depressed	Fluctuating
Motivation in cognitive tests	Poor – gives up easily	Usually tries their best
Awareness of cognitive problems	Highlights problems	Tries to conceal problems

Clinical feature	Depressive pseudodementia	Dementia
Progress of cognitive impairment	Fluctuating	Constant cognitive decline
Pattern of condition severity	Typically worse in morning	Typically worse later in the day
Other depressive symptoms	Invariably present	Sometimes present

On the subject of mood disorders, it is also worth mentioning bipolar disorder. Individuals with this condition experience periods of depression, though these are interspersed with periods of elevated mood known as *hypomania* or *mania*. In these latter states, there may be a subjective state of elation or euphoria, increased energy and activity, and a reduced need for sleep. Overtalkativeness can occur, and sometimes there are uncharacteristic risky or impulsive behaviours. Cognitive problems may occur when someone with bipolar disorder is in a depressed state, but also when their mood is elevated – in the latter state, they tend to be easily distracted and have difficulty staying on task. In addition, there seems to be a chronic damaging effect of having the condition meaning that with time, even when the person is well from a mood perspective, there may be residual cognitive deficits.

Anxiety and stress

As with depression, there is an association between anxiety and dementia. Dementia increases the risk of anxiety developing, and anxiety can portend the development of dementia. It has also been shown that those with MCI who have high levels of anxiety are 135 per cent more likely to develop dementia than those without anxiety.

Anxiety and stress can have a significant effect on cognition. The impact of these symptoms is readily understandable to most of us, as we all experience periods when we struggle to recall things because of a stressful situation. People under stress may report feeling 'paralysed' and 'unable to think'. Whatever it is that we forget may well come back to us when our anxiousness has settled, however.

The most prominent aspects of cognition affected by anxiety appear to be that of selective attention and working memory.

The impact of *chronic stress* is also worth considering. This state is often associated with abnormally high levels of the hormone cortisol, as well as other inflammatory chemicals. In one study, high levels of cortisol were correlated with faster cognitive decline in individuals with high levels of beta-amyloid in their brains. Inflammation is one possible underlying cause of Alzheimer's disease, so this may explain the connection between stress and dementia.

Research into the relationship between stress and cognitive impairment is complicated by difficulties around defining what 'stress' actually is, and by its close association with other problems, such as depression, that may also cause cognitive problems.

Symptoms of anxiety are generally divided into the physical and the psychological domains:

- *Physical symptoms* may include muscle tension, headaches, a racing heart or experience of palpitations, chest tightness, hot and cold flushes, rapid breathing, feeling agitated and 'wound up', and the experience of a lump in the throat or butterflies in the stomach. Nausea may occur, as might diarrhoea.
- *Psychological symptoms* include fear, excessive worry, obsessional rumination (thinking over the same stressful thing again and again, and having difficulty stopping doing so), irritability and catastrophising (imagining the worst-case scenario).

Psychotic illness

Although psychotic illnesses such as schizophrenia are relatively uncommon compared to depression and anxiety, it is important to recognise that they are a potential factor in cognitive impairment. The most problematic cognitive decline in those with a psychotic illness comes about where it is a chronic condition that has developed relatively early in life and has exerted a long-term damaging effect on nerve cells. Areas of cognition impacted by these conditions include working memory, long-term memory and processing speed – these roughly correlate with poorly functioning frontal and temporal areas of the brain. Apathy and poor motivation also often accompany these conditions, and can create an impression of cognitive impairment that is worse than the reality.

Symptoms of a psychotic illness may include *delusions* (firmly held beliefs that are incorrect) and *hallucinations* (such as hearing or seeing things that do not exist). Some of these psychotic symptoms can occur as part of dementia itself, though their nature is often a little different to those in people experiencing an independent psychotic illness. Chapter 11 describes these in more detail.

In summary

With all these psychological conditions, the *sequence* in which they and the cognitive symptoms emerge is important to clarify, as this may help us identify the primary problem. If the initial symptoms are those of anxiety and/or depression, it is more likely these are the primary issue, whereas if cognitive deficits occur first, dementia is more likely. Yet as we have seen, psychological symptoms can be the first manifestation of dementia, so it can be tricky to draw a definitive conclusion. In such cases, it is important to address the psychological symptoms (through psychological therapy or with medications) regardless of whether they are the cause or effect of dementia.

Depression, anxiety and psychotic illnesses are all readily treatable illnesses. Whether or not there are obvious cognitive problems, whoever has symptoms suggestive of these conditions should seek help from family, friends, their local GP or, if need be, a psychologist or psychiatrist. Treatment may be as simple as resolving some external problems in one's life, or implementing lifestyle changes that are known to be beneficial. Or it may involve engaging with a psychologist for structured psychological therapy. In some cases, the use of medications can be very helpful in alleviating symptoms.

See the Appendix for helpful resources on psychological illness and its treatment.

Physical conditions that may cause cognitive impairment

Given that the majority of people with cognitive problems are in their more senior years, it is not surprising that many of them have a range of other physical health problems. These may cause cognitive impairment in someone without dementia, or may exacerbate the problem in those with dementia.

In those with a moderately severe dementia, even the most minor disturbance in bodily functioning may cause significant changes in cognition. In nursing homes, urinary tract infections can be rife, and they're probably one of the most common reasons for an acute decline in cognition in someone with a known dementia. Even constipation can cause this problem for some.

A number of physical health conditions are known to be associated with cognitive problems even when dementia is not present. The more common examples, along with some of their associated symptoms, are listed below.

- *Low thyroid function.* Symptoms include weight gain, dry skin, lethargy, constipation and slow pulse rate.
- *Obstructive sleep apnoea.* Symptoms include weight gain, snoring, periods of not breathing overnight, headache and profound daytime fatigue.
- *Diabetes (uncontrolled).* Symptoms include dry mouth, increased thirst, increased urination, slow healing, dizziness, drowsiness, blurred vision, headache, trembling and light-headedness.
- *Low blood sodium.* Symptoms include weakness, fatigue, headache, nausea, vomiting, irritability, muscle cramps, drowsiness and seizures.
- *Renal (kidney) impairment.* Symptoms include nausea, vomiting, loss of appetite, change in pattern of urination, muscle twitches, itching, swelling of feet and ankles, breathlessness and high blood pressure.
- *Hepatic (liver) impairment.* Symptoms include yellowing of skin, upper abdominal pain, abdominal swelling, nausea, vomiting, malaise and sleepiness.
- *Parathyroid disease.* Symptoms include bone pain, thinning hair, fatigue and headache.
- *Multiple sclerosis.* Symptoms include fatigue, loss of vision, episodes of urinary incontinence, areas of sensory change (such as pins and needles or pain) and poor balance.

- *Low levels of B vitamins.* Symptoms include weakness; fatigue; swollen tongue; numbness or tingling in hands, legs or feet; and unsteadiness.

When assessing cognitive changes, it is important to investigate the possibility of all these conditions before concluding the presence of a dementia. The good news is that many of them can be identified with standard medical investigations, and most are amenable to treatment.

Perimenopause

Menopause, or the cessation of menstruation, classically occurs in women between the ages of 45 and 55, though it may occur in someone in her thirties, or conversely not develop until someone is in her sixties.

Perimenopause refers to the period leading up to menopause. This may last for a number of years before menstruation finally ceases, and is characterised by a number of well-recognised physical symptoms. These include hot flashes, night sweats, irregular periods, sleep problems, vaginal dryness and mood symptoms. These latter psychological problems may occur in up to 20 per cent of perimenopausal women.

Perimenopause and menopause are driven by hormonal changes – chiefly, alterations in the level of oestrogen in the body. This hormone rises and falls unpredictably during perimenopause, and this oscillation may account for the cognitive problems seen in some people experiencing the condition. Oestrogen is known to influence function in many brain regions responsible for cognition, including the hippocampus, the prefrontal cortex and subcortical structures.

Oestrogen promotes health in brain cells and optimises effective transmission between them. When there is a loss of oestrogen, the nerve cells suffer and cognitive problems may develop. This may be compounded by the impact of the perimenopausal mood changes noted above. Cortisol levels may spike during perimenopause, which can also have a deleterious effect on cognition.

The cognitive changes that can occur during perimenopause

are generally mild – similar in severity to those seen in MCI. There may be problems with memory, executive function and speed of thinking. Unlike MCI, however, there is not a greater conversion to dementia than seen in the general population.

Although blood tests may help identify whether someone is perimenopausal, the levels of hormones may vary considerably over time and so a single test may be unhelpful. Sequential testing can address this issue, though many doctors do not routinely use blood tests, instead basing their thoughts on the symptoms and signs of the individual.

The symptoms of menopause are sometimes treated with hormone replacement therapy (HRT). See Chapter 4 for a discussion of the impact of HRT on cognition; the bottom line is that the evidence is not conclusive. As a general rule, HRT is not recommended for treatment of these cognitive symptoms (though it may be appropriate for other reasons).

Head injury

The brain, especially in the elderly and in alcoholics, is susceptible to traumatic injuries, which most commonly occur in these groups due to falls. A patient's history will usually give a hint that this may be a problem, but not always. Although the cognitive problems associated with head injuries are usually acute (sudden) after the injury itself, they can be delayed for days, weeks or even months. This is particularly the case in those with underlying cognitive problems, when the *change* in cognition is less obvious.

The usual mechanism of damage is via a *haemorrhage*, or abnormal bleeding inside the skull or brain. Head injuries are generally detectable using structural brain scans (see Chapter 13) and may require surgical intervention.

A particular condition called *chronic traumatic encephalopathy* is known to result from repeated head injuries, and can predispose an individual to dementia. Classically it occurs in those who regularly engage in contact sports such as rugby. The cognitive signs may develop many years after the initial injuries. (This condition is the subject of the 2015 Will Smith film *Concussion*, about the plight of professional football players in the United States.)

Medications that may cause cognitive impairment

In tandem with the increased prevalence of physical health problems in the elderly, the use of medications also increases substantially. Although the majority of these medications may be required for optimal treatment of other health conditions, some can cause significant cognitive difficulties.

Analgesics (pain relievers) are one category of medications where problems may arise. Thankfully, paracetamol (Panadol), the most commonly used form of oral pain relief, has no proven deleterious effect on cognition when taken in prescribed amounts. Likewise, anti-inflammatories such as ibuprofen are probably unlikely to cause cognitive harm.

The problem with pain relief comes when more potent agents are required. Most commonly, this includes the *opioid analgesics* – those based on the opium poppy, such as codeine, morphine, oxycodone, pethidine, buprenorphine and fentanyl. These can cause increased confusion both directly and by inducing sedation in an individual. Less commonly used medications, often reserved for neuropathic pain (examples include pregabalin and gabapentin) may also cause some decline in cognition. Chapter 19 provides more detail about the use of these medications by those with dementia.

Other medications cause cognitive problems by interfering with the brain's *cholinergic system*. Disruption of this system underpins the cognitive symptoms of Alzheimer's disease. Individual medications that interfere with the cholinergic system – so-called *anticholinergics* – may be reasonably well tolerated, but there are many commonly used medications that may have this effect, and the cumulative impact can be significant. Medications with anticholinergic properties include certain antidepressants, medications for Parkinson's disease, medications for urinary incontinence, medications to regulate blood pressure, anticonvulsants and some diuretics. Antihistamine medications, commonly given to help with sinus issues and allergies, can also be problematic.

In theory, any medication that has a sedative effect can also cause cognitive problems. Many psychiatric medications may have this effect. Medications in the same group as diazepam (benzodiazepines) can cause problems, as can sedating antidepressants and certain antipsychotics.

In the initial assessment of someone with cognitive problems, it is imperative that an accurate medication history is obtained. Sometimes alternative medications can be employed that may not be such a problem from a cognitive perspective. If there is no alternative, it comes down to weighing up the pros and cons of someone remaining on the medication, and trying to clarify how great an effect it is having on their cognition.

The following table sets out some commonly used medications that may cause cognitive impairment, either acutely or with chronic administration. It should be noted that for a number of these medications, different studies demonstrate different results – some studies raise concern and others seem to dismiss the risk. Nonetheless if you are taking any of these medications, their potential deleterious cognitive effect needs to be borne in mind.

Psychiatric medications	Benzodiazepines – e.g. diazepam, oxazepam, lorazepam, alprazolam, nitrazepam
	Sleep-inducing medications – e.g. temazepam, zopiclone, zolpidem
	Some antidepressants – e.g. paroxetine, tricyclic medications such as amitriptyline, clomipramine, dothiepin, doxepin, nortriptyline
	Some antipsychotics – e.g. chlorpromazine, olanzapine, quetiapine
	Lithium
Neurological medications	Some Parkinson's medications – e.g. benztropine, levodopa, amantadine, tolcapone
	Some anticonvulsants – e.g. carbamazepine, phenytoin, phenobarbital, topiramate, pregabalin
Antihistamines	Chlorpheniramine, cetirizine and diphenhydramine
Cardiovascular drugs	Warfarin, atenolol, metoprolol and digoxin

Drugs used to treat acid reflux	Ranitidine, cimetidine, omeprazole and esomeprazole
Steroids	Prednisolone and methylprednisolone
Painkillers	Primarily opiate-derived substances – codeine, morphine, buprenorphine and oxycodone
Drugs used for urinary incontinence	Tolterodine and oxybutynin

Commonly used medications that may cause cognitive impairment.

Statins

It is worth discussing statins – medications used to reduce blood cholesterol – in a little more detail as there has been a great deal of discussion in the media about their relationship with cognitive impairment, including dementia.

In the early 2000s, a couple of influential studies raised concerns about the negative short-term effect that statin therapy had on cognition, noting that people on these medications appeared not to improve on tasks of learning as compared to those on a placebo. Further studies have disputed these findings, however. Some believe there may be a subset of individuals who have a particular genetic make-up that renders them vulnerable to this negative effect of statins, possibly due to their inability to neutralise free radicals produced by the mitochondria – the energy centres of the cells. One study found that those who report other side effects when taking statins – muscle pain and weakness – may be more at risk of cognitive impairment, and that higher-potency drugs such as rosuvastatin (sold as Crestor) and atorvastatin (sold as Lipitor) carry more risk.

There has also been some concern that reducing cholesterol may itself cause cognitive problems, as cholesterol is one of the core components of myelin, the insulating material on nerve cells that allows for the effective transmission of messages.

Despite these concerns, however, there is reason to suppose that statins may in fact prevent cognitive impairment. By lowering cholesterol, we reduce one of the risk factors for vascular disease, and this should help cognitively. Statins may also have direct anti-inflammatory effects on the brain. Some observational studies have supported this idea of cognitive protection. However, a comprehensive 2016 review suggested there is not enough evidence to support this idea if statins are started when someone is in their sixties or seventies. Importantly, the review commented that if statins are started during midlife, the situation may be different – but this appears not to have been greatly studied.

The bottom line with statins is that the evidence remains unclear, and it is therefore hard to give definitive advice. Cognitive health is only one potential ramification of their use. Heart health is another important factor to consider, and the evidence does suggest that statins help reduce the risk of heart attacks and strokes. All these things need to be taken into account.

The problem of delirium

Delirium is also known as an *acute confusional state*; as this term suggests, it presents with an acute (over hours or days) change in a person's mental state. It classically has a fluctuating course, meaning that the affected individual may at times be reasonably lucid, though at other times appear very confused and disoriented. There is also usually an abnormal fluctuation in the level of consciousness, with the person having unexpected periods of drowsiness interspersed with more alert moments or even periods of *hypervigilance* (a state of hyper-alertness, sometimes coupled with anxiety or paranoid thinking).

The most obvious cognitive problem in delirium is that of poor attention – the patient may have great difficulty focusing on the conversation, and their responses to questions may be rambling and tangential. Disorientation – not being aware of where you are, or what the time, day or date is – is also a frequent, though non-specific, symptom.

Delirium can also be associated with changes in psychological and behavioural functioning – a person may experience or show anxiety, mood changes, agitation, aggression or psychotic symptoms. It is a condition that requires urgent medical attention.

Delirium should be considered in anyone who shows the above symptoms, whether or not they have an underlying dementia.

Those with dementia are more at risk of developing delirium owing to reduced cognitive reserve, and it is important to consider when someone known to have dementia has a sudden worsening of cognitive problems, as this may suggest a treatable condition. It can be due to multiple causes, many of which are identical to the physical health problems and medication causes noted above. Often it may be due to multiple causes, none of which alone may have caused the problem, but which cumulatively will do so. For example, someone with a urinary tract infection may also be taking opiate-derived painkillers.

Although delirium is quite distinct from dementia in most cases, one type of dementia – that associated with Lewy bodies – has a symptom profile that can be very similar. This type of dementia therefore always needs to be borne in mind when classic delirium-type symptoms develop.

The following table sets out the major distinctions between delirium and dementia.

Clinical feature	Delirium	Dementia
Onset	Sudden and abrupt; often at twilight	Insidious/slow
Alertness	Often impaired and fluctuating	Usually unaffected
Course	Short. Daily fluctuations in symptoms. Worse at night; in darkness; upon waking.	Long, with less fluctuation. Symptoms progressive but stable over time.
Duration	Hours to weeks, or longer if untreated	Months to years

How to tell the difference between delirium and dementia.

The next chapter explores pathological syndromes of cognitive impairment that do not reach the threshold for dementia.

6

More than Ageing, but Not Dementia

- There are recognised conditions in which cognition is impaired beyond that expected for age, but which do not represent dementia. These are known as subjective cognitive impairment (SCI) and mild cognitive impairment (MCI).

- Both SCI and MCI may improve over time, though there is an increased risk of developing dementia with these conditions, especially with MCI.

- The emphasis with both SCI and MCI is on remaining physically healthy, eating well and remaining cognitively and socially active.

- Signs of SCI and MCI should be discussed with your doctor and closely monitored.

It is not uncommon for me to see individuals who complain of memory or other cognitive problems that are beyond what one would expect from ageing alone, but who can lead normal lives. They do not have dementia as they are not functionally impaired, but nor is their situation 'normal'. Researchers have come up with two broad categories for this type of problem: *subjective cognitive impairment* (SCI) and *mild cognitive impairment* (MCI). Neither is attributable to psychological, medication related or physical problems, but psychological symptoms can accompany them.

Subjective cognitive impairment

SCI, also known as *subjective cognitive decline* or *subjective memory complaints*, is a state in which the person reports a decline in cognitive (or other) abilities, though these deficits are not able to be demonstrated on recognised cognitive tests. Symptoms of SCI may include:

- Word-finding difficulties
- Increasing forgetfulness
- Losing one's train of thought
- Mood changes, especially depression
- Feeling anxious or overwhelmed when having to plan or make decisions.

SCI is a common phenomenon and its implications are unclear. Certain studies suggest that it may be a very early (pre-clinical) stage of dementia, with evidence that its presence predicts conversion to Alzheimer's disease and is associated with an increased amyloid build-up in the brain.

SCI may just as readily not develop into dementia, however, and indeed may improve, so if you have symptoms of this condition, you should be alert but not alarmed. SCI warrants further discussion with a medical practitioner (who may perform some basic investigations), but, once determined, the best course of action may simply be watchful waiting.

At the same time, I always advise individuals with SCI to take note of the BRAINSCAN factors noted in Chapter 3: lead a physically active life; ensure vascular risk factors, such as high blood pressure and cholesterol, are well controlled; consume a healthy diet; and engage in cognitively and socially stimulating activities.

Mild cognitive impairment

MCI, also known as a *minor neurocognitive disorder*, is a state of cognitive difficulty exceeding that seen in normal ageing, but lacking the functional impact or other features of dementia.

To qualify for this 'diagnosis', the person must report cognitive problems, or have someone who knows them well report these concerns. As opposed to SCI, however, the cognitive deficits must also be apparent in formal cognitive testing (usually performed by a health practitioner involved in their care). As opposed to dementia, the individual must be able to generally perform their usual daily activities, although there may be a subtle deterioration in their ability to complete more complex tasks; this sometimes manifests as a deterioration in work performance.

Two types of MCI are generally recognised:

- *Amnestic MCI* – in which memory impairment is the most prominent symptom. This tends to be the most common type of MCI, and if it develops into dementia, it is most commonly of Alzheimer's type.
- *Non-amnestic MCI* – which is characterised by impairment of other cognitive skills, such as language. This type of MCI may more readily evolve into an alternative dementia, such as dementia with Lewy bodies, vascular dementia or frontotemporal dementia.

The association between MCI and dementia is more robust than that for SCI and dementia; it has been estimated that 10–15 per cent of those with MCI go on to develop dementia each year. This compares to only 1–2 per cent of older people in the general population who develop dementia each year. Considered another way, the risk of developing any type of dementia if MCI is present is three to five times greater than if it is absent.

It is not known why some individuals with MCI go on to develop dementia and some do not. Certain factors do seem to increase the risk, however. These include older age, increased severity of cognitive impairment and certain biomarkers (see Chapter 13). Amnestic MCI has also been shown to be more likely to progress into dementia than non-amnestic MCI. Amyloid deposition in the brain (detected on brain scans) may also occur with MCI, and its presence also heightens the risk of developing dementia in the future.

It should also be noted that it is far from inevitable that having MCI means you will develop dementia in the future; some individuals with MCI may become cognitively normal with time. The 10–15 per cent annual conversion rate to dementia noted above means of course that 85–90 per cent of people with MCI do not develop dementia each year.

A finding of MCI should prompt further investigation, including blood tests, urine tests and possibly neuroimaging (CT or MRI scans). Various conditions may mimic MCI, and these need to be excluded. These include psychological problems such as depression or anxiety, the side effects of certain medications, various physical health problems and nutritional deficiencies. These are discussed in the previous chapter. Subtle changes in personality or psychological functioning (such as increased anxiety, frustration or mood changes) may also occur as part of MCI, however, and it can be difficult to determine what came first.

Predictably, there has been a great deal of interest in recognising and potentially treating MCI before it develops into dementia. Unfortunately, however, there is no conclusive evidence that the medications we use to treat cognitive problems in dementia are effective in MCI. Most studies have shown little benefit and have also noted problematic side effects. Research continues apace, though, and it is hoped the future will bring more helpful pharmacological strategies for treating MCI and lessening the chances of it evolving into dementia.

Much like with SCI, interventions in someone who has developed MCI tend to be focused on optimising nutrition, getting more physical exercise (progressive weight training has been associated with reduced shrinkage of the medial temporal area of the brain, where the hippocampus resides) and promoting socialisation. Optimising risk factors for vascular disease is important, and management of psychological stress may also protect against conversion from MCI to dementia. See Chapters 2 and 3 for more information about these.

There is also some evidence that cognitive training may be beneficial, though the generalisability of improvements on cognitive tasks is not clear. Individuals may improve in the specific cognitive tasks they are trained in, but it is not certain whether this translates to noticeable everyday improvements in daily function. Again, see Chapter 3 for more information on this topic.

There are a number of other reasons it is important to recognise the presence of MCI. Doing so, and knowing that there is an increased risk of dementia, allows an individual to create an action plan for the future. This may involve optimising their physical and psychological health, evaluating their support systems and ensuring that their legal affairs (such as their substitute decision-maker paperwork and will) are in good order (see Chapter 21 for more information about these aspects.) It should also be recognised that MCI is associated with a greater risk of developing psychiatric problems such as depression and anxiety, and it is important that these are dealt with.

Once an individual has been determined to have MCI, it is critical that they receive regular monitoring, at a minimum by their GP. This increases the chance that any signs of dementia will be recognised quickly. Early recognition is important for a number of reasons, including that the medications currently available for cognitive enhancement tend to work best in the early stages of dementia.

7

Dementia Defined

- Dementia is a description, not a diagnosis, and is sometimes referred to as a major neurocognitive disorder.
- There are many types of dementia, of which Alzheimer's disease is the most common. Vascular dementia, dementia with Lewy bodies, alcohol-related dementia and subcortical dementias account for the vast majority of the other cases.
- Dementia is characterised by cognitive and other symptoms that represent a change from a previous level of ability, that get worse as time passes, and that cause impairment of daily functioning.
- Memory loss is not always the first or most prominent symptom of dementia. The symptoms depend on the location of the underlying damage.
- Dementia may cause a number of behavioural and psychological symptoms. These are often the most challenging part of the condition, but treatments are available.

Although there has perhaps been some positive shift in the last few years, I regularly observe the misconception among patients and their carers that Alzheimer's disease and dementia are the same thing. This confusion is understandable – the two words often appear synonymously in the popular press, and Alzheimer's disease is one type of dementia. But it is important to be clear about the distinction between the two.

Dementia is not one thing. Nor is it a diagnosis in and of itself. Just like cancer, in order to make a diagnosis you need to know the underlying *cause* of the problem. 'Dementia' is really no more than a word we use to describe a collection of irreversible and worsening symptoms that occur as a consequence of a particular brain disease – it is an umbrella term. So when you hear of someone having 'dementia' it does not tell you what is causing their disease, just that they have certain symptoms.

Causes of dementia

Dementia has a number of causes. There are over a hundred, in fact, though a handful account for the vast majority of cases. The cause (and therefore the specific diagnosis) of a dementia is determined by two things: what is going wrong with the brain tissue (the pathology) and the location of this pathology in the brain.

The best known and most common cause of dementia is *Alzheimer's disease*. Other common causes include *vascular dementia* (which is related to poor blood supply), *frontotemporal dementia* and *dementia with Lewy bodies*. *Alcohol-related dementia* is also not uncommon, as is dementia associated with other neurological diseases such as *Parkinson's disease* or *Huntington's disease*. These different causes of dementia will be explored in more detail in the following chapters.

When it comes to *late-onset dementia* (occurring in those aged 65 or over), Alzheimer's disease accounts for about two thirds of cases. The majority of other cases are related to vascular disease and possibly dementia with Lewy bodies, though in my experience frontotemporal dementia, dementia due to Parkinson's disease and alcohol-related dementia are not uncommon.

When dementia affects those under 65 – so-called *early-onset dementia* (or *younger onset dementia*) – Alzheimer's disease remains the most common cause, accounting for about 30 per cent of cases. Twenty per cent are due to vascular disease and frontotemporal dementia, while alcohol-related dementia and dementia with Lewy bodies account for about 10 per cent each. In Australia in 2020, there are thought to be about 28,000 people with early-onset dementia (of all types). This equates to about 4–5 per cent of all cases. Early-onset dementia is often misdiagnosed – as depression, for instance, or some other mental health disorder. It may take some time before it is correctly identified. This may be in part due to the unexpected nature of a dementia occurring at a younger age.

Common features of dementia

The symptoms of dementia vary according to the cause. Some individuals, like those with Alzheimer's disease, often initially present with short-term memory impairment. Language or behavioural changes may be the first problem in frontotemporal dementia. Vascular dementia symptoms are related to which part of the brain has impaired blood supply. Despite these differences, however, a number of elements are common to the different dementia types.

First of all, the symptoms must represent a *change* from what someone used to be like. Everyone's brain enters old age with intrinsic strengths and weaknesses. I, for instance, have always been awful at remembering names. If that's the only cognitive problem I have when I'm older then it will not be a change for me, and therefore would not indicate that I am developing dementia, even though I might be impaired compared to some. If my wife developed the same problem, I might be more concerned, though, as she has an uncanny ability to recall the names of almost everyone we meet. What really counts when considering the possibility of dementia is not the deficit itself, but whether the deficit indicates a decline from a previous level of ability.

There must also be progression of impairment – that is, a continued decline of abilities as time passes. There are exceptions to this – someone whose dementia relates to alcohol use may improve if they stop drinking alcohol, for example – but a progressive deterioration in skills and function is by far the most common pattern.

Exclusion of other causes of cognitive impairment is also required if we are to have certainty about dementia being present. As we saw in Chapter 5, numerous psychological and physical conditions can cause symptoms that are reminiscent of dementia, and these need to be ruled out.

The time frame is also a relevant factor. There are numerous causes of cognitive impairment, especially in those most at risk – the elderly – and the nature of their onset can be a guide as to whether a dementia is present or whether something else is going on. In general, a sudden change in thinking is unlikely to be related solely to dementia; if this occurs, it should lead one to consider other diagnoses, such as delirium (see Chapter 5). Although there are some exceptions – certain types of vascular dementia, for instance – dementia normally develops gradually. The fact that individuals are often not diagnosed until the condition is quite advanced supports this: the changes can be so slow to develop that they go unnoticed for some time.

Over the last decade, there have been a number of revisions and refinements to the criteria for dementia in general, and also in relation to its specific subtypes. In part this is due to our increased understanding of the diseases that cause the condition. The most recent edition of the globally recognised *Diagnostic and Statistical Manual of Mental Disorders* (known as the DSM-5) uses an alternative but equivalent term for dementia: 'major neurocognitive disorder'. This term was adopted in part to reduce the stigma associated with the term 'dementia', as well as to differentiate it from a *minor neurocognitive disorder* (also known as *mild cognitive impairment*). As we saw in Chapter 6, one of the key distinctions between the two conditions is that in dementia the cognitive problems are severe enough to cause an impairment of daily function.

Cognitive skills affected by dementia

In Chapter 1 we looked at the cognitive functions of the healthy brain, all of which can be affected by dementia. One of the changes in the most recent DSM-5 is that memory impairment no longer has to be present for a diagnosis to be made. Instead it lists six *cognitive domains*, all of which may be affected to differing degrees.

Complex attention

This relates to our ability to attend (or pay attention) to what is going on around us (stimuli), and incorporates sustaining attention (on one thing), dividing attention (between more than one stimulus at one time) and being selective in our attention (filtering out irrelevant stimuli). Attention also influences the speed at which we can process information around us.

In everyday life, deficits in attention may lead to someone not following conversations, mislaying objects or having difficulty staying on task or remaining focused. These problems may be especially noticeable in environments where there are multiple competing stimuli (such as noises from the TV, more than one conversation or lots of people).

Learning and memory

This incorporates working/short-term memory and long-term memory. Problems in this area may manifest as repetitiveness in conversation, forgetfulness and disorientation. Awareness of time and dates may be impaired, medications and appointments forgotten, and everyday objects frequently misplaced.

Language

This involves both expressive language skills (the ability to express what we are thinking) and receptive language skills (the ability to understand what is being said to us). Individuals with difficulties may be vague in their word use, such as by referring to objects as 'that thing', or they may talk around something as they cannot remember the appropriate word. They may also substitute the wrong word for one they have forgotten. They may not understand the words being said to them, and may therefore be unable to follow instructions.

Executive ability

Individuals with difficulties in this area may struggle with more complicated tasks, or those that require sequencing (doing things in a certain order) or multiple steps/elements. Planning becomes difficult and disorganisation often results. Poor judgement may arise. The ability to prepare a cooked meal is an example of a task that is contingent on executive function, as is the management of financial affairs. Loss of motivation and drive may occur with impaired executive function, and some may experience difficulty thinking in more abstract ways.

Social cognition

This relates to our ability to act in a socially appropriate manner, to recognise the emotions of others and to moderate our behaviours and basic drives. Self-care and grooming may deteriorate if there are problems in this area, and there can be a significant impact on the individual's ability to interact with others in the expected fashion. Social cognition is closely associated with executive ability.

Perceptual/motor/visual perception/praxis

This pertains to our ability to correctly interpret visual stimuli, to know where various body parts are in space and to coordinate ourselves accordingly. Deficits in this domain may mean individuals have trouble handling kitchen utensils, showering, getting dressed, walking and driving.

In the early stages of dementia, it is unusual for all domains to be affected equally, and different types of dementia cause different problems. As the damage spreads throughout the brain tissue, however, the impact becomes more global, and in the latter stages of most types of dementia, most cognitive skills show a degree of impairment.

Other symptoms and signs of dementia

In addition to the cognitive changes above, dementia is often associated with other symptoms and signs, including those affecting our physical function. We will discuss many of these in Part Two of this book.

Mood changes, anxiety and even psychotic features commonly occur at different stages of the disease; some may be due to the process of adjusting to the knowledge that one has a progressive and terminal disease, although the damage wrought by the underlying disease process also contributes. Changes in behaviour are also common. These non-cognitive symptoms are referred to collectively as *behavioural and psychological symptoms of dementia* (BPSD). Recognition, understanding and treatment of these is again a particular focus in Part Two.

In the next chapter we will look at the two most common types of dementia: Alzheimer's disease and vascular dementia.

8

Alzheimer's Disease and Vascular Dementia

- Alzheimer's disease is the most common type of dementia.

- Accumulation of abnormal proteins – beta-amyloid and tau – in the brain is associated with Alzheimer's disease. Damage to the nerve cells in the brain and decreased connectivity cause symptoms.

- The typical early symptom of Alzheimer's disease is the inability to form new memories. As the disease spreads throughout the brain, other cognitive symptoms occur.

- There are non-modifiable and modifiable risk factors for dementia. The way we live our lives many years before dementia is likely to occur can have a significant effect on our risk of developing dementia.

- Behavioural and psychological symptoms of dementia are common and are often the aspects that cause the most difficulty for carers.

- Vascular dementia is caused by disruption to the blood supply to the brain and can develop suddenly or gradually. The symptoms of vascular dementia depend on which area of the brain has been damaged.

- There are numerous risk factors for vascular dementia, although many can be reduced by being physically active and eating well.

Time for a coffee. This chapter and the next detail the commoner forms of dementia: Alzheimer's disease, vascular dementia, frontotemporal dementia, alcohol-related dementia and subcortical dementias. These are probably the most information-heavy chapters in the book, but they provide valuable information about the medical causes of the symptoms many of those with dementia experience.

Alzheimer's disease

Alzheimer's disease is a *neurodegenerative* condition, which means that the brain cells of those with the condition become damaged or die, leading to the reduction or loss of brain function. The degeneration is progressive, meaning the damage gets worse with time. In the following pages we will discuss the possible causes of Alzheimer's, its signs and symptoms, its genetics and how the disease progresses. First, though, let's understand how prevalent Alzheimer's is, and what its major risk factors are.

How common is dementia due to Alzheimer's disease?
Alzheimer's disease is the most common cause of dementia. It is generally divided into *early-onset* and *late-onset*, depending on whether the symptoms and signs develop before or after the age of 65. The large majority of cases are late-onset.

From a population perspective, the worldwide prevalence for dementia due to Alzheimer's disease is 3.9 per cent for people aged 60 and over, though there is considerable variation in different countries (rates in Africa are 1.6 per cent, for instance, while in the United States they are 6.4 per cent). In Australia, the quoted figure is 8.8 per cent, though this includes other types of dementia.

Risk factors for developing dementia due to Alzheimer's disease
As with any medical condition, there are *risk factors* for dementia due to Alzheimer's disease – things that increase our chances of developing the condition – and *protective factors*, which reduce the chances. It is helpful to consider risk factors as being either *modifiable* or *unmodifiable*.

Unmodifiable risk factors

These are risk factors that we cannot change. By far the biggest risk factor for Alzheimer's disease is advancing age. Estimates of age-related risk vary from study to study, though in our mid to late sixties the chance of developing dementia due to Alzheimer's disease is probably somewhere between 2 per cent and 5 per cent. This risk then doubles approximately every five to six years, meaning that by the time we reach our late eighties, and certainly our nineties, there may be a 30–50 per cent chance of developing the condition. The risk of developing dementia due to Alzheimer's disease rises exponentially with age, especially for women. Given that the average lifespan in Australia is a little over 82 years, this is a sobering thought.

Genetic vulnerability is the other major unmodifiable risk factor for Alzheimer's disease, and is discussed a little later in this chapter. Being female also increases the risk of developing dementia due to Alzheimer's disease. This has historically been thought to be related to the fact that women live longer, but there may be other factors at play. A Stanford University study from 2014 showed that the risk associated with having a particular variant of a gene (APOE4) was significantly higher for women than men. We also know that heart health and vascular health are risk factors for developing Alzheimer's disease, and there is a belief that men who have avoided death from these conditions (being more at risk in this respect than women) and who have survived into old age may have particularly favourable vascular health, which is therefore protective against developing dementia due to Alzheimer's disease.

Modifiable risk factors

Much of the research conducted on modifiable risk factors for dementia has not been specific to Alzheimer's disease, and there are therefore some limitations to our knowledge about this specific issue. Nonetheless, recognising that most dementia arises later in life and that Alzheimer's disease is by far the commonest cause, it is fair to assume that the more general research into modifiable risk factors holds true for Alzheimer's disease. As we saw in Chapter 3, approximately 35 per cent of the risk factors for dementia are thought to be things we can change. This is encouraging, as it means that around a third of new cases of the condition might be prevented if we address these risks.

The following is a list of factors that have been associated with an increased risk of Alzheimer's disease:

- Vascular factors (related to blood supply), including
  ° Midlife high blood pressure
  ° High blood cholesterol
  ° Midlife obesity
  ° Diabetes
  ° Cerebrovascular disease
  ° Smoking
- Nutritional factors
  ° Deficiencies in folate, vitamin B12 and antioxidants (vitamins A, D, E and C)
- Other factors
  ° Traumatic head injuries (especially repeated, such as those related to sports)
  ° Poor sleep
  ° Exposure to toxins
  ° Depression, especially chronic and occurring later in life
  ° Chronic psychological stress
  ° Poor hearing.

This is unlikely to be an exhaustive list of risk factors, and more are likely to be uncovered with time. An interesting 2020 study, for instance, raised the possibility that living close to a main road is a risk factor. Although pollution may intuitively be blamed for this, this specific measure was not correlated with the risk of developing dementia due to Alzheimer's disease. This may be a facet of the study design, of course, but clearly there are many unanswered questions about the risk factors that may exist.

Indigenous Australians
Across a number of health domains, Indigenous Australians are more at risk than non-Indigenous Australians. These include for kidney

disease, respiratory disease, diabetes and cardiovascular disease. It has also been shown that the rates of dementia are increased in Indigenous communities; in one study looking at the Northern Territory, the estimated prevalence of dementia for Indigenous people over 45 was more than three times the rate seen in non-Indigenous people. Alzheimer's disease was considered the most common type of dementia, followed by vascular dementia. Another study looking at Indigenous communities in the Kimberley showed an even greater discrepancy: an estimated fivefold increase in risk compared to non-Indigenous communities. Being male, being a smoker, having suffered a head injury or stroke, and having received a poor education were identified as risk factors. Regardless of the exact figures, the findings are sobering and provide yet more impetus for Australia to 'close the gap'.

Protective factors

Factors that may reduce our risk of developing Alzheimer's disease include the following:

- Psychosocial factors
  - High educational attainment
  - Bilingualism or polylingualism (speaking at least two languages)
  - Mentally stimulating activities
  - Social activity and an enriched social network
  - Physical activity
- Vascular factors
  - Use of blood pressure-lowering medications
- Nutritional factors
  - Light to moderate alcohol consumption
  - Fish and vegetable consumption
  - Mediterranean diet
  - MIND diet.

There may be other protective factors too. A Finnish study in 2016 suggested that enjoying a regular sauna may reduce the risk of dementia. Saunas are known to have cardiovascular benefits, and this may explain the relationship – though the relaxing nature of such a pastime may also contribute.

The homocysteine conundrum

Homocysteine is an amino acid (a compound that forms the building blocks of proteins). It occurs naturally in our bodies and can be measured through a blood test. High levels of homocysteine have been associated with vascular problems and Alzheimer's disease. High concentrations also seem to be associated with low levels of certain B vitamins (folate, B6 and B12) – vitamins usually derived from what we eat. Increasing our intake of these B vitamins results in homocysteine levels dropping back to normal. (See Chapter 3 for an outline of helpful dietary sources of B vitamins.)

Interest in homocysteine as a predictor of and target for Alzheimer's has waxed and waned over the last 20 years, though a recent international consensus statement argued that it is important to consider it as a modifiable risk factor for the condition. Studies so far looking at supplementation with B vitamins – a logical treatment – have been plagued by methodological problems, however, and more research is needed to clarify this issue.

Anaesthesia

I am often asked about the interface between dementia and general anaesthesia. It is a pertinent issue, as age increases both the risk of dementia and the need to have surgical procedures that would require anaesthesia.

What is clear is that anaesthesia can exacerbate cognitive problems in those with underlying dementia, whatever its cause. The chances of developing delirium (an acute confusional state; see Chapter 5) after an anaesthetic are higher in those with pre-existing dementia. Delirium may linger for weeks to months in some individuals, and for a number this may in fact be the event that unmasks the presence of dementia.

What is less certain is whether anaesthesia increases the risk of dementia developing in the first place. Studies on animals have shown that certain anaesthetic drugs increase the rate at which beta-amyloid forms in the brain, but this may not be relevant to humans. Studies looking at the association between anaesthesia and dementia in humans have failed to demonstrate conclusively that the former causes the latter. The question has not therefore been comprehensively answered.

Clearly, any decision regarding surgery and anaesthesia has to consider a number of factors, many of which are not related to cognition. It is important to discuss all the risks and benefits of any surgery with your doctor.

The genetics of Alzheimer's disease

When I tell someone I think they have dementia due to Alzheimer's disease, they or their relatives often become concerned about what this means for family members. In particular, they worry about the chances of them developing the condition. This is something that can be quite difficult to estimate, though the age of onset of the dementia is a key influencing factor when it comes to genetic risk.

Early-onset dementia is defined as having an onset before the age of 65, and accounts for 5–10 per cent of known cases of dementia due to Alzheimer's disease. The risk of relatives developing dementia is considerably higher for early-onset dementia than for later-onset dementias. When early-onset dementia occurs as part of a genetic pattern in a family – that is, when it's inherited – it is sometimes referred to as *familial dementia* or *early-onset familial Alzheimer's disease*. It may be related more to the overproduction of amyloid in the brain than to the problem with reduced breakdown of amyloid seen in late-onset dementia. The role of amyloid in Alzheimer's disease is discussed in greater detail later in this chapter. Some cases can also occur 'out of the blue', with no familial link – these are known as *sporadic* cases.

Familial or inherited early-onset dementia is usually caused by an inherited change in one of three genes (segments of DNA housed in cellular structures called chromosomes). These genes include:

- The amyloid precursor protein gene on chromosome 21
- The presenilin 1 gene on chromosome 14
- The presenilin 2 gene on chromosome 1.

Mutations in these genes affect either the structure of a protein called amyloid precursor protein or the way in which it is processed (cleaved). This leads to the accumulation of beta-amyloid in the brain – something that is associated with Alzheimer's disease. Again, these substances are discussed in more detail below.

We receive genes from our parents – one copy from our mother and one from our father. Individuals with one or two copies of the faulty genes referred to above will go on to develop Alzheimer's disease: the faulty gene is dominant and therefore overrides the influence of a normal gene. A child of someone with one faulty gene has a 50 per cent chance of developing the disease. This is dependent on whether they receive the normal or faulty copy from their parent. This is the usual case and assumes the other parent does not have the rare gene mutation. If one parent has two faulty genes, it is inevitable that their child will also get the faulty gene and develop the condition at some stage, assuming they live long enough. If both parents have one faulty copy each, there is a 75 per cent chance the child will receive it and develop dementia.

Late-onset dementia is considerably less genetically influenced than early-onset dementia, with environmental and lifestyle factors playing an equal or bigger role, though one genetic risk factor has been determined: the apolipoprotein E (APOE) gene.

This gene is located on chromosome 19 and may come in different forms (called *alleles*): APOE2, APOE3 and APOE4. Which form you have influences your genetic risk of developing Alzheimer's disease:

- APOE2 is quite rare, but possibly confers some protection against Alzheimer's; if dementia does occur, it tends to occur at a later stage than in someone with APOE4.
- APOE3 tends to be neutral and therefore does not influence risk greatly.
- The APOE4 allele seems to increase the risk of developing Alzheimer's disease, and may result in it occurring at an earlier age. The more APOE4 alleles one has (zero, one or two), the greater the risk. With one copy, the risk is doubled. With two

APOE4 alleles, the chances of developing Alzheimer's are increased by a factor of 12 to 15. The risk seems greater for women than men.

It is important to note that APOE4 is only a risk factor, and a person may have two APOE4 alleles and not develop dementia due to Alzheimer's disease. Also, only half the people with this condition have the APOE4 allele. A blood test can be taken to ascertain what APOE alleles a person has, but this tends to be used more in research than in clinical practice, at least in Australia.

The risk of someone aged 65 developing dementia due to Alzheimer's disease by age 87 if they have a first-degree relative (parent, sibling or child) with the condition has been shown to increase fivefold. Another way of looking at the statistics is that if a close relative (a parent or sibling) has the condition, the risk of developing it yourself is 30 per cent higher than the risk in someone who has no close relative with the disease.

In practice, genetic testing to determine whether you have one of the mutations above is not usually recommended or undertaken unless there is a strong family history of early-onset dementia.

What causes Alzheimer's disease?

This remains an unanswered question, though there are a number of theories. The most common are the *amyloid cascade hypothesis* and the *tau hypothesis*, as well as theories involving *inflammation* and *oxidative stress*. Let's look at these in more detail:

Amyloid and tau

Alzheimer's disease was named after Alois Alzheimer, a German psychiatrist and neuropathologist active in the late 19th and early 20th centuries. In 1906 he reported on an 'unusual disease of the cerebral cortex' in a 55-year-old woman who presented with memory loss, hallucinations and disorientation. Examination of this lady's brain after her death showed a number of abnormalities, including thinning of the cortex, the presence of *plaques* normally only seen in the brains of the elderly, and *neurofibrillary tangles* – other abnormal clumps of protein – that had not previously been identified. These features are still considered very relevant to a diagnosis of Alzheimer's disease today.

Strictly speaking, Alzheimer's disease remains a *pathological* or *histological* diagnosis, meaning it is dependent on finding these abnormal structures – the plaques and neurofibrillary tangles – in the brain. These are only visible using a microscope and require us to biopsy the brain, something that, for obvious reason, is not usually done until after death. In life, therefore, we generally refer to someone having *probable* Alzheimer's disease (in which the classical clinical features are present), or *possible* Alzheimer's disease (where the presentation is not typical or usual, though no other clear cause is considered likely).

The plaques are composed of beta-amyloid, a type of protein that accumulates in clumps both outside of and between nerve cells. Beta-amyloid is formed when a larger protein, *amyloid precursor protein*, which sits in the wall of nerve cells, is cleaved (broken down) in a particular way. The exact function of beta-amyloid and why it accumulates remains unclear. Some researchers believe it has a protective function, and that it is produced in response to toxic processes such as inflammation or infection. Regardless, these clumps have been hypothesised to cause dysfunction in a number of ways, including by promoting inflammation themselves. Their accumulation also seems to precipitate the formation of tau, another type of protein, and interferes with the normal transmission of messages between nerve cells. Cell death is associated with the accumulation of beta-amyloid. All these processes lead to the symptoms and signs of dementia. It is still not confirmed, however, whether these plaques are the actual cause of or a product of Alzheimer's disease.

It should also be noted that amyloid may accumulate in the brain many decades before the clinical symptoms of dementia appear, and its presence does not mean that dementia is inevitable. Ageing alone can lead to the accumulation of beta-amyloid in the brain – especially from the fifth decade onwards – but this does not always result in significant cognitive decline. In Alzheimer's disease, however, the accumulation tends to be greater, and from an early stage is classically located in certain locations: in the hippocampus, deep within the medial temporal lobe of the brain, and in particular parts of the cortex associated with thinking. With the spread of amyloid to different parts of the brain as time goes on, the symptoms and signs of Alzheimer's increase. The degree to which the plaque burden correlates with the severity of dementia is actually quite weak, however, leading a number of researchers to question the so-called amyloid hypothesis of Alzheimer's disease.

Neurofibrillary tangles are made up of *tau*. This is found in nerve cells, rather than outside of them, and ordinarily stabilises tiny channels (*microtubules*) within nerve cells that allow effective passage of nutrients and molecules from one end to another. In Alzheimer's disease, the chemistry of tau is altered, leading to it pairing with other threads of tau to form a tangle. Once in this formation, tau is no longer able to play its stabilising role and the microtubules disintegrate, resulting in impaired function of the nerve cell.

Like amyloid plaques, tangles also tend to gather initially in the medial temporal lobes, including in the hippocampi. Similarly, with time, they spread to other parts of the brain.

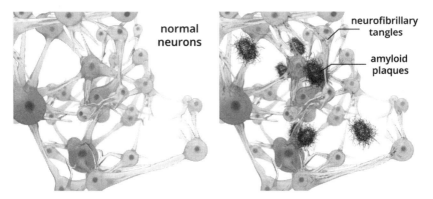

Amyloid plaques and neurofibrillary tangles accumulate in the brain in Alzheimer's disease.

There is still debate about the relative contribution that tangles and plaques make to the signs and symptoms of Alzheimer's disease, but the net result of their presence is reduced function of neurons, death of neurons and disrupted communication between them. All of this leads to the clinical manifestations of the disease.

Inflammation and oxidative stress

These two processes are intimately linked, with oxidative stress considered to be a major cause of chronic inflammation. This inflammation has been associated with a number of chronic age-related diseases, including cancer, diabetes and cardiovascular disease, in a process creatively termed *inflammaging*.

In part owing to the failure of therapies that target beta-amyloid and tau, questions have been raised over other possible factors, including inflammation, that might contribute to the risk of Alzheimer's disease. Pathological studies have shown that the brains of people with this neurodegenerative condition show changes in certain types of supporting nerve cells – glial cells – that suggest inflammation is occurring. Unfortunately, however, the use of drugs that suppress this neuroinflammation has not yielded promising results, suggesting that the relationship between inflammation and Alzheimer's disease is not straightforward.

Oxidative stress occurs when there is a disturbance in the balance between *free radicals* (molecules of oxygen produced by numerous processes in the body) and *antioxidants*, which ordinarily 'mop up' the free radicals – a good thing, as free radicals damage various tissues in the body. It has been shown that Alzheimer's disease is highly associated with oxidative stress, and that there is a connection between beta-amyloid and oxidative stress. As with inflammation, however, oxidative stress is only part of the picture. Numerous substances have purported antioxidant properties (examples include vitamins C and E, omega 3 fatty acids and ginkgo biloba), though the evidence that they are helpful in changing the course of Alzheimer's disease is not compelling (see Chapter 4 for more information).

One optimistic aspect of the hypothesis that inflammation and oxidative stress may underpin Alzheimer's, however, is that both processes may be amenable to dietary interventions and other lifestyle choices that reduce inflammation (see Chapter 3).

Other theories

There are some other theories about the cause of Alzheimer's disease, including one involving the immune system: at one stage an immunotherapy drug called AN-1792 seemed to hold great promise for preventing Alzheimer's disease, though when it was trialled in humans a number developed encephalitis (inflammation of the brain) and the trial had to be ceased. Brain insulin resistance (the inability of cells to respond to insulin by taking glucose – sugar – out of the bloodstream) is also gaining increasing attention in the research field. Other aspects of the endocrine (hormone) system are being investigated too. The gut – including both our oral and intestinal microbiome – may also be involved, possibly through inflammatory mechanisms.

It seems likely that no one theory alone will account for Alzheimer's disease, and these theories are on the whole not mutually exclusive. It is probable that a large combination of factors is at play.

Disruption to the cholinergic system

As discussed in Chapter 1, for nerve cells to do their job properly they need to transmit messages from one end to the other, and then on to an adjacent nerve cell. In order to pass the message on from one cell to another, a chemical messenger must leave the end of one nerve cell, move through the gap between the nerve cells (the synapse) and reach the neighbouring nerve cell endings on the other side of the gap.

Many types of chemicals are involved in this process – they are collectively known as *neurotransmitters* – but in the context of the cognitive impairment seen in Alzheimer's disease, one of these, *acetylcholine*, is particularly relevant. This neurotransmitter is the key messenger in a type of brain circuitry known as the *cholinergic system*. Disruption of the cholinergic system is considered to be pivotal in the development of the cognitive problems seen in Alzheimer's disease.

As we age, the amount of acetylcholine between our nerve cells decreases, and this process is amplified in Alzheimer's disease. In fact, it has been estimated that the levels can drop by 90 per cent in this type of dementia. This effectively leads to a breakdown in communication between the nerve cells – and without adequate communication, the system fails, giving us the symptoms of the disease. It is rather like a car's engine running without enough oil.

Three out of the four medications we use to treat Alzheimer's disease work by increasing the levels of acetylcholine in the cleft. They do this indirectly, by inhibiting (reducing) the action of an enzyme called cholinesterase, which normally breaks acetylcholine down in the cleft and reduces how much is available. These medications are thus called *cholinesterase inhibitors*; we'll discuss their use in Chapter 15.

Disruption to other neurotransmitter systems
As well as the cholinergic system, Alzheimer's disease also causes changes to numerous other neurotransmitters, including glutamate (the target for another cognitive-enhancing drug, memantine), dopamine (relevant for changes in movement and some psychological symptoms), serotonin and noradrenaline (also very relevant to psychological changes), and gamma-aminobutyric acid (a neurotransmitter that in the adult brain has a calming effect). This in part explains the various non-cognitive symptoms that can occur in Alzheimer's disease.

Biomarkers and brain changes in Alzheimer's disease
In the last decade, there have been revisions and refinements made to the diagnosis of Alzheimer's disease, and at least two sets of well-recognised criteria have been developed – one by the National Institute on Aging–Alzheimer's Association in the United States and the other by the International Working Group for Alzheimer's Disease. Although these criteria vary a little, both recognise the importance of *biomarkers* in addition to clinical symptoms. These biomarkers include structural brain changes, the presence of amyloid and tau on brain scans, and the presence of amyloid or tau in the cerebrospinal fluid. Some of these biomarkers can be detected before there are even any symptoms or signs of Alzheimer's disease, allowing the recognition of so-called *pre-clinical Alzheimer's disease*. This has important research and clinical implications.

The most common early structural brain abnormality in Alzheimer's disease is atrophy (shrinkage). This can be detected via CT scans or MRI scans. The former has the advantage of being cheap and quick, though may not show adequate detail in many cases. An

MRI brain scan, however, can detect relatively subtle shrinkage in the hippocampi and temporal lobes, which is characteristic of late-onset Alzheimer's disease.

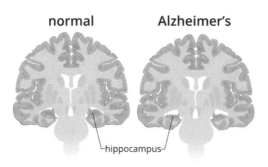

A coronal slice (front to back) of the brain; the hippocampus, a critical structure for learning, starts to shrink early in late-onset Alzheimer's disease.

It should be noted that such changes can occur to some extent in people who do not have cognitive problems or dementia. Similarly, normal brain scans do not exclude the possibility of dementia; such scans are only one part of the diagnostic puzzle.

If Alzheimer's disease occurs before the age of 65 (early-onset), the hippocampi may not be so overtly shrunken. A more frequent abnormality may be shrinkage of the posterior (back) part of the cortex. This is known as *posterior cortical atrophy*, and is discussed a little later in the chapter.

There are also brain scans available in Australia that detect the presence of amyloid long before the development of a clinical dementia. These are special types of PET scans, a form of imaging discussed in more detail in Chapter 13. These are not yet routinely used, except in research. Although these scans can be helpful in some cases, at this stage they tend to be neither sensitive nor specific enough to be of general use in clinical practice. A 2014 review showed that only 1 per cent of people with a negative amyloid scan (that is, one that did not show a significant amount of amyloid) went on to develop dementia, but that 28 per cent of those with a positive scan (one showing amyloid) did not develop dementia. Scanning for tau is also available and may hold more promise than amyloid imaging when it comes to predicting future brain changes associated with Alzheimer's disease. A 2020 study also showed that a blood test for tau (ptau-217) may be as good as PET imaging in predicting the future development of the disease, though more research is needed to clarify its use in everyday practice.

Signs and symptoms of Alzheimer's disease

The early hallmark feature of late-onset Alzheimer's dementia is short-term memory loss and the inability to form new memories. It is the damage to the hippocampus and medial temporal lobe noted above that causes this problem. The impaired function of these structures means information that has been registered by the brain is not properly encoded, sorted or sent on to the cortex for storage. Information therefore cannot be recalled after it has disappeared from our conscious awareness, even after a relatively short period of time. In day-to-day life, this may present as forgetfulness (of conversations, medications, appointments and so on), repetitiveness in conversation, disorientation or frequently losing possessions.

As we saw in Chapter 1, different parts of the brain are responsible for short-term and long-term memories. The latter, which have 'moved on' from the hippocampus after being recalled (remembered and brought to mind) lots of times, are less vulnerable to the erosive effects of dementia. Memories from a long time ago have been laid down before the damage to the hippocampus began, and have been recalled many more times than more recent ones. This process of recalling and remembering memories consolidates the circuitry underpinning the memory, strengthening it. Hence, there is a so-called *temporal gradient* to memory loss: the more recently formed memories (especially what has happened in the last few hours to days) are the first to go. In short, it's last in, first out.

As the tangles and plaques spread to other parts of the brain, so too does the neuronal damage. From the temporal lobes, the disease may spread forward to the frontal lobes, upwards and outwards to the parietal lobes, and then backwards to the occipital lobes. As the pathology spreads, other cognitive skills may become affected.

The involvement of the parietal lobe may involve difficulties related to visual and spatial skills – these are not uncommon early signs of dementia due to Alzheimer's disease: drawing and writing may become affected, for instance, as may everyday activities that require physical manipulation of objects, such as getting dressed and operating machinery. This is known as *apraxia*. Calculation may be affected. Understanding language may become difficult – so-called *receptive aphasia*.

Symptoms and signs of frontal-lobe involvement include difficulties sustaining attention, poor planning and judgement, social impropriety, increased impulsivity, mood changes and apathy (loss of drive). The person may have difficulties finding the right word. More complex cognitive tasks – those involving multiple steps and manipulation of information – become increasingly difficult to complete. Changes in personality may begin to show. *Expressive aphasia* – the inability to use language effectively – may also occur.

As the occipital lobe becomes involved, specific problems with visual awareness and recognition may emerge. Individuals may struggle to work out what is in front of them.

Damage to a number of different areas may cause other symptoms, including *agnosia*, which is an inability to recognise familiar objects or people – either by sight, sound or touch. This symptom can lead to failure to recognise family or friends, and to impairment of everyday tasks such as getting dressed or using cutlery.

Remembering that the nerve cells in the brain are all part of one large circuit, it is evident that the problems in Alzheimer's disease, along with most other dementias, are problems of impaired connectivity. This has led to some describing Alzheimer's disease as a 'disconnection syndrome'.

Damage to various other parts of the brain can cause both psychological disturbance and changes in physical function. We'll discuss these in some detail later in the book.

Both the cognitive and non-cognitive symptoms and signs of Alzheimer's disease classically worsen toward the end of the day, a term often referred to as *sundowning*.

The progression of Alzheimer's disease

Alzheimer's usually develops *insidiously* (slowly) and progresses gradually. In my experience, however, the progression is not necessarily linear and there may be periods of apparent stability followed by periods of more precipitous decline. It should be noted that a very abrupt decline should always cause us to question whether something else is going on that is exacerbating the cognitive impairment, such as a urinary tract infection, but it's possible for a *subacute* decline, over a period of weeks to months, simply to be part of the dementia.

Complicating things, there may be fluctuations in someone's level of lucidity from day to day or week to week. Carers of people with Alzheimer's disease often remark on unexpected periods of awareness and lucidity, against a background of more general confusion.

The experience of dementia due to Alzheimer's disease can be divided into stages – from mild (early stage) to moderate (middle stage) to severe (late stage). There is considerable variation in the rate at which individuals progress through these stages, and the specific symptoms they may encounter in each.

In the initial phase, although there may be overt problems with memory and forgetfulness, someone with Alzheimer's may still be able to function reasonably independently. They may drive without incident, continue to work, and be able to maintain good social relationships. There may be periods of transient disorientation, however, and they may struggle to remember, for instance, where they parked their car. Unfamiliar routines and environments may exacerbate their cognitive symptoms and increase their stress. Apathy and a loss of drive may be evident, and a loss of confidence may cause them to withdraw from normal activities. Anxiety is not uncommon, with the awareness that something is not right. More complex tasks may be difficult to achieve and frustration may result, sometimes presenting as irritability.

As the middle stage is reached, a person may have increasing difficulties performing daily tasks, especially ones that are more cognitively complex, such as managing their finances. People in this phase of the illness still often retain important details about their life, and their memories of remote events are often quite clear. Others around them may observe words being muddled, as well as increasing frustration and irritability (in part due to their awareness of their impaired abilities). There may be increasing problems with attention and judgement, meaning that risky behaviours such as leaving the gas oven on may become more prominent. Changes in behaviour, such as a decline in personal hygiene, are not uncommon. Repetitiveness may become more pronounced, and the names of familiar people may be forgotten. Routine tasks can become harder to perform as the person passes through this stage. There may be more persistent and severe difficulties in orientation – not knowing where they are or what day it is – and problems with maintaining continence. Sleep patterns may be affected, and individuals can become quite restless overnight. In some cases, wandering may occur.

Other behavioural and psychological symptoms may become problematic in the middle stages, including suspiciousness and repetitive behaviours like hand-wringing. Individuals may ask the same question multiple times. Anxiety can become more prominent and may be associated with a fear of abandonment, exacerbated by their awareness of their impaired ability to cope by themselves. This stage of the illness tends to be the longest of the three and may last many years.

The late stage of Alzheimer's disease is characterised by severe symptoms. Those in this stage of the illness may not be able to respond appropriately to their environment and may struggle to carry on a conversation. There may be increasing loss of bodily function; incontinence is more usual than not. Mobility deteriorates and language function may greatly diminish – both the ability to articulate concerns and to understand what is being said to them. At this stage, it is highly likely that the individual will need help with bathing and even feeding, and permanent care is often required. There may also be increasing medical problems associated with the decline in physical function, including pneumonia, chewing and swallowing difficulties, and pressure sores. Yet some of the psychological distress that may have accompanied the earlier stages may spontaneously disappear as this third stage is reached.

The average span of time from diagnosis to death is between three and seven to eight years, though this depends on the stage at which the dementia is diagnosed. Often, individuals do not receive a diagnosis until they are in the more moderate to severe stages of the illness. This may seem surprising, but can occur for a number of reasons:

- The erroneous belief that nothing can be done for dementia
- The existence of 'denial' (not being psychologically ready to accept a diagnosis)
- A fear of being diagnosed
- A reluctance to being seen by someone who can make the diagnosis
- The assumption that cognitive decline is just part of ageing.

The progression of Alzheimer's disease may vary greatly from person to person, and it can be quite hard to predict the rate of change.

I am often asked how quickly someone experiencing dementia due to Alzheimer's disease will deteriorate. This is hard to answer, and is often influenced by other physical health problems that may develop. I do emphasise, though, that if the condition is picked up early, they may be able to enjoy a number of years of relatively good function and preserved quality of life.

Certain factors seem to be associated with a more rapid decline, unfortunately. These include being younger at the age of onset and having had more education (though this latter factor seems to protect against dementia developing in the first place). Vascular disease – high blood pressure and high cholesterol – has been shown to hasten the progression. In the study that determined this, however, diabetes, which we might predict would increase the rate of decline, did the opposite, for reasons that remain unclear. Malnutrition is also associated with a faster deterioration.

Behavioural disturbance and psychotic symptoms also seem to be associated with a greater rate of decline. Such phenomena reflect the fact that Alzheimer's disease, and indeed dementia more generally, affects not only cognition but other aspects of our being. The term *behavioural and psychological symptoms of dementia* (BPSD) is a useful one when discussing these very relevant issues. BPSD are common, and often are the most problematic area of dementia, though effective interventions are available. See Chapter 16 for further discussion of this important topic.

Atypical Alzheimer's disease

Our discussion so far of the nature and symptoms of Alzheimer's relates to the typical presentation of the disease. But there are also less common forms of the disease, known as *atypical Alzheimer's disease*, where the initial damage tends not to be in the hippocampus, and therefore short-term memory loss is not an early sign. About 5 per cent of late-onset dementia cases fall into this category, but atypical dementias account for up to a third of early-onset dementia cases.

The most common atypical variants are:

- *Posterior cortical atrophy.* The damage here is primarily to the back part of the brain, including the occipital lobe. This leads to problems with processing visual information and impairment of spatial awareness. In day-to-day life, a person may have difficulty recognising objects or reading, experience incoordination, or have trouble judging distances. It is often misdiagnosed as anxiety or depression, and is a not-uncommon form of early-onset Alzheimer's disease. The well-known author Terry Pratchett, who passed away in 2015, had this condition.
- *Logopenic aphasia.* With its name deriving from the Greek for 'word poverty' and 'speechless', this condition is characterised by early loss of language skills. Individuals may speak fluently though use the wrong words, or they may begin to stutter and stumble their words. This is the result of damage to parts of the left temporal lobe and parietal lobe.
- *Frontal variant Alzheimer's disease.* The damage here is to the frontal lobes, and the initial presenting symptoms and signs are generally executive problems and changes in behaviour and personality.

Vascular dementia

Vascular dementia is the second-most common cause of dementia, after Alzheimer's disease. It is estimated that between 1 and 4 per cent of people aged 65 have this condition, with the risk doubling every five to ten years after that. Men tend to be more at risk of vascular dementia than women, especially in those under 75.

This is probably because men are more likely to have vascular disease in general.

What is vascular disease?

The term 'vascular' derives from the Latin term *vasculum*, meaning 'vessel'. In the context of medicine, it refers to the system of veins, arteries and other vessels that supply blood to different parts of our body, including our brain. Different prefixes are attached to the word that relate to which part of our body the blood is supplied: *cardio*vascular means the blood supply to and from the heart, for instance, while *cerebro*vascular refers to the brain's blood supply.

Vascular dementia is a catch-all term for dementia caused primarily by problems with blood supply, the result of damage caused by cerebrovascular or cardiovascular disease. Without an adequate blood supply, oxygen and vital nutrients cannot reach parts of the brain, and nerve cells are exquisitely sensitive to changes in oxygenation. This damage can be created by obstruction of a blood vessel (by a blood clot, for example), in which case it is called an *infarct*. If this is temporary it may result in a TIA, or *transient ischaemic attack*. The resulting symptoms may be very brief, and officially should last no more than 24 hours. A TIA is also sometimes called a 'mini stroke'. Blood can also escape from the vessel into adjacent brain tissue, causing a haemorrhage. Both these events in the brain may cause what we commonly refer to as a *stroke* or, in medical parlance, a *cerebrovascular accident*.

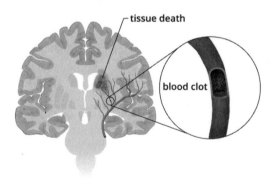

Vascular disease results in the death of brain tissue.

There are a number of subtypes of vascular dementia, of which the most common are:

- *Multi-infarct dementia.* This type of dementia is caused by numerous small strokes in the brain causing damage. The strokes often affect isolated areas of the brain, and so the symptoms may be limited to one side of the body and may affect only a few cognitive functions. Each small stroke may be 'silent' – that is, it may not cause obvious symptoms by itself – but cumulatively these strokes can result in marked cognitive impairment. Multi-infarct dementia is probably the most common type of vascular dementia.
- *Single-infarct dementia.* Although not all strokes result in dementia, if the stroke is large enough or affects particular locations it can result in dementia. This is more likely to be the case when the stroke affects the left hemisphere of the brain or if it affects the hippocampus, which is critical for memory storage and encoding.
- *CADASIL.* This stands for *cerebral autosomal dominant arteriopathy with subcortical infarct and leukoencephalopathy* – hence the acronym! It is a subtype of multi-infarct dementia, and is a hereditary disorder caused by defects in a specific gene (Notch3). The result is a dementia state, at times associated with features of migraine and mood disturbance. Unusually, it often begins in one's twenties, thirties or forties, and may go undiagnosed for many years.
- Dementia related to *severe low blood pressure.*
- *Brain haemorrhage*, resulting in a sudden onset of symptoms.
- *Autoimmune conditions* such as systemic lupus erythematosus. These may cause inflammation of the blood vessels.
- *Inflammatory disease* such as temporal arteritis (inflammation of the temporal arteries).

Binswanger's disease

This is a specific type of vascular dementia that affects the *subcortical areas* of the brain. It is caused by multiple tiny areas of damage to the brain's white matter (the axons of the nerve cells). Its risk factors are similar to those for other types of vascular dementia. Unlike other types of vascular dementia, however, it may begin early in life, from late in the fourth decade. It becomes more severe with age and has a characteristic appearance on CT and MRI scans of the brain.

Like other subcortical disease (see Chapter 9), the symptoms of Binswanger's reflect problems with executive function, including prominent difficulties with planning, organisation and attention. One very notable feature is that of *psychomotor slowness* – a slowing of thinking and movement. Mood and personality changes may occur, as may problems with bladder control and clumsiness.

There is no cure for Binswanger's disease, though its psychological symptoms can be treated. Optimising vascular risk factors in general may slow the progression of the condition.

Mixed dementia

It should be noted that there is good evidence that the pathology of Alzheimer's disease may increase the risk of stroke (and therefore vascular dementia), and that stroke and vascular disease increase the risk of developing Alzheimer's disease. This may result in a so-called *mixed dementia*. The same beta-amyloid protein associated with Alzheimer's disease can also lodge itself in the walls of blood vessels, in a condition known as *cerebral amyloid angiopathy*. This effectively weakens the vessels, and brain haemorrhages may result. The relationship between the two diseases is not well understood, but inflammation may be a common underpinning. When one problem – either Alzheimer's changes or vascular changes – damages the brain, our brain reserve is depleted, meaning it is more sensitive to other damage.

Risk factors

The risk factors for vascular dementia are the risk factors for vascular disease in general:

- Hypertension (high blood pressure)
- Atrial fibrillation (a disordered heart rhythm)
- High cholesterol in midlife
- Diabetes and pre-diabetes

- Obesity
- Poor diet (particularly one high in saturated fat)
- A sedentary lifestyle
- Smoking
- A family history of vascular disease (either cardiovascular or cerebrovascular).

It is not surprising, given the above, that leading a physically active life and eating well are protective against vascular dementia. As we saw in Chapter 3, it is important to address vascular risk factors early on, at least from midlife.

Clinical features of vascular dementia

The onset of dementia associated with vascular disease is related to the underlying disease process. Single-infarct dementia results in a sudden-onset dementia (one of the few instances of this), whereas multi-infarct dementia is usually gradual in onset and more akin to that seen in Alzheimer's disease. Which symptoms are experienced depends on where the stroke damage has occurred. The progression of symptoms is often described as 'step-wise' – things may get suddenly worse after a further cerebrovascular event; this is in contrast to Alzheimer's disease, which progresses gradually.

Memory problems may occur, although short-term memory is not as prominently affected as in Alzheimer's disease. One distinguishing factor is that cueing (providing clues or prompts about what has been forgotten) can often help the person remember what it is that they have forgotten. This probably has something to do with the fact that vascular dementia causes a problem with retrieval rather than acquisition of memories – the information usually 'goes in' but may take some coaxing to be recalled. In Alzheimer's disease, the information does not 'go in' in the first place due to a faulty hippocampus, and so there is nothing to be recalled, even with cueing. Other cognitive functions commonly affected in vascular dementia include concentration, language (both expressive and receptive language) and executive problems.

There may be other features of a stroke that do not involve cognition, such as slurred speech, sudden weakness, numbness and poor coordination (especially down one side of the body), sudden loss of vision or one-sided facial drooping. These symptoms do not typically occur in Alzheimer's disease. There may also be changes in gait (walking), problems with balance and, in some cases, a slowing of thinking and movement.

Vascular dementia is thought to be more likely to result in mood changes than Alzheimer's disease, particularly a depressed mood, as well as anxiety and irritability. There may also be changes to the person's underlying personality – they may change from being respectful and reserved to uncaring and dismissive. Interestingly, in my experience, these changes in personality are not always a bad thing. I have seen people who by nature have been morose and pessimistic becoming more carefree and optimistic. *Apathy* is a not-uncommon symptom of vascular dementia; it denotes a state of reduced interest and drive that is unrelated to depression.

The prognosis for vascular dementia is generally worse than for Alzheimer's disease, possibly related to the fact that there are usually other medical comorbidities (such as heart disease), although strict control of vascular risk factors can help in slowing down progression.

In the next chapter, we'll look at the other common types of dementia.

9

Frontotemporal, Alcohol-related and Subcortical Dementias

- Frontotemporal dementia preferentially affects the frontal and temporal lobes of the brain. Symptoms typically involve changes in language and/or behaviour. Some types involve the subcortex and cause movement problems.

- Unlike in Alzheimer's disease, memory is relatively preserved in early frontotemporal dementia.

- Alcohol is a toxic substance, though when taken infrequently and in moderation it may not be overly harmful to the brain. Excessive long-term use is undoubtedly associated with dementia, however.

- Alcohol-related dementia causes symptoms of executive dysfunction and memory impairment through damage to the hippocampi and frontal lobes. Symptoms may improve with prolonged abstinence from alcohol.

- Dementias involving the subcortex relatively early on include Parkinson's disease dementia, dementia with Lewy bodies, Huntington's disease dementia, HIV-related dementia and some types of vascular dementia.

- Subcortical dementia classically presents with slowing of movement and thinking, abnormal movements, and prominent mood and other psychological symptoms.

Although the following causes of dementia make up the notable minority, they highlight the different ways in which dementia can present. They pose their own challenges and are important to recognise.

Frontotemporal dementia

Also known as *frontotemporal lobar degeneration*, this type of dementia preferentially affects the frontal lobes and/or the temporal lobes of the brain. Frontotemporal dementia is not one disease, but a number of diseases grouped together owing to their involvement of common parts of the brain, and their similar symptoms and signs. Frontotemporal dementia differs from Alzheimer's disease in a number of ways; perhaps the most obvious is that, in the early stages, memory function is relatively spared. It is considerably less common than Alzheimer's disease, accounting for under 3 per cent of dementias in those over 65, although it's responsible for 10 per cent of dementias in those under 65.

Most cases of frontotemporal dementia are sporadic, meaning they occur without an obvious family history, although 10–15 per cent of cases are inherited. Language variants are less likely to be inherited than behavioural variants.

The historical recognition of frontotemporal dementia as a disease actually preceded that of Alzheimer's disease: it was first described by neurologist Arnold Pick in the late 19th century. Dr Pick identified the abnormal presence of clumps of protein in nerve cells, and these became known as *Pick cells*. For many decades after this, frontotemporal dementia was often referred to as *Pick's disease*, though in the last few decades the definition of frontotemporal dementia has evolved greatly. Pick's disease is now considered one of many presentations of frontotemporal dementia.

The classification of frontotemporal dementia is a somewhat controversial topic, and there is also considerable overlap between different types. Unlike in Alzheimer's disease, the hippocampus is not typically affected in frontotemporal dementia, at least early on, accounting for the relative sparing of pure memory function in the early stages of the illness. There is also an association between frontotemporal dementia and a number of other neurological conditions, including motor neurone disease and parkinsonism.

Classification of frontotemporal dementia by symptom and location

Frontotemporal dementia can be divided into two clinical types, depending on the dominant symptoms experienced. These are known as the *behavioural variant* and the *language variant*.

Behavioural variant frontotemporal dementia

This is also known as the *frontal variant* frontotemporal dementia and tends to occur when the initial damage is to the frontal lobe. This results in certain early behavioural and personality changes:

- Poor insight into the condition is a notable symptom. This can be a challenge clinically, as not infrequently the condition occurs when the individual experiencing the condition is still working but does not recognise the problems they have.
- A loss of social awareness is also a common finding in frontal variant frontotemporal dementia; individuals may come across as uncaring, unempathetic, insensitive or rude.
- There may be inappropriate behaviours, including disinhibition (a loss of normal social restraint, as well as a disregard for social conventions), aggression, apathy, hoarding and compulsions.
- Anxiety may be evident early on, as may mood changes. Obsessionality and rigid behaviours and attitudes may also occur, though impulsivity (acting without thinking) is also not uncommon.
- Dietary changes may occur – typically a preference for sweet foods or a general increase in consumption of food. Individuals may not act appropriately in regard to eating, and may take food from others.
- Humour may become more childish or fatuous, with a disregard for the offence it may cause (a phenomenon known as *Witzelsucht*, literally 'joking addiction' in German).

Damage to the frontal lobe also causes *executive dysfunction*, or the loss of a number of cognitive skills that are required for more complex cognitive tasks. This includes the ability to set goals, to solve problems, to do things in sequence and to organise oneself.

Language variant frontotemporal dementia

This second variant preferentially affects the temporal lobe, though typically the *anterior* (forwardmost) part, rather than the *medial* part affected by Alzheimer's disease. In this variant the primary symptom is loss of language function. It is also known as *primary progressive aphasia*. This is sometimes further divided into *semantic dementia* and *progressive non-fluent aphasia*.

- Semantic dementia is characterised by the ability to speak fluently/clearly, though with impaired ability to find the right word for the situation. Semantic memory relates to our understanding of meanings, words and ideas. Impairment of this often results in the wrong word being used (*paraphasia*) – either one that sounds similar (*phonological* or *phonemic paraphasia* – such as 'pike' for 'pipe') or one that is incorrect but similar in meaning (*semantic* or *verbal paraphasia* – such as 'wife' for 'husband'). Individuals with semantic dementia may also talk around a point as a compensatory mechanism (*circumlocution*).
- Progressive non–fluent aphasia, by contrast, causes a breakdown in speech production. Speech may be generally slowed, halting or stuttering and filled with hesitation. There may be associated frustration due to an awareness of the errors and the extra effort required to create speech. As the disease progresses, the amount of speech output becomes reduced – sentences may become simpler – and individuals may become entirely mute.

The behavioural variant of frontotemporal dementia is thought to be four times as common as the language variant. As frontotemporal lobar degeneration progresses, however, there is less distinction between the two types, and both language and behavioural changes may coexist.

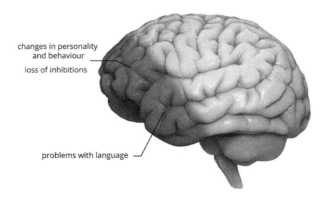

changes in personality
and behaviour

loss of inhibitions

problems with language

The symptoms of frontotemporal dementia correspond to the areas that are damaged in the brain.

Classification of frontotemporal dementia by histology

Frontotemporal dementia has also been classified according to the underlying *histological* findings – that is, those seen on examination of the brain tissue using a microscope – and, in particular, according to the types of abnormal proteins that are absent or present. This is a complicated and expanding field of research, though there are three broad categories.

Those with tau present

This is the same protein that has been implicated in Alzheimer's disease, with the Pick cells mentioned earlier having tau as a chief constituent. These are known as *tau-positive frontotemporal dementia syndromes*. There are three commonly recognised subtypes of tau-positive frontotemporal dementia:

- *Pick's disease.* Mentioned earlier, this manifests as the behavioural variant of frontotemporal dementia.
- *Corticobasal degeneration.* This disease involves the cortex but also the subcortex, and in particular the basal ganglia. The typical symptoms resemble those seen in Parkinson's disease: rigidity of muscles, slowed movements, tremor, shuffling gait and a stooped posture. It tends to affect one side of the body and can result in a phenomenon known as *alien limb syndrome*, where the limbs seem to move of their own

accord. Speech is often halting, like that seen in *progressive non-fluent aphasia*, and swallowing difficulties can occur. From a cognitive perspective, language, visuospatial and executive skills are affected earlier than memory.

- *Progressive supranuclear palsy*. This condition also presents with features of parkinsonism due to the involvement of the basal ganglia, but it involves other areas as well, such as the cortex and brainstem. It is the involvement of the brainstem, which houses the nerves responsible for eye movements, that leads to the most distinguishing feature of the disease: abnormal eye movements and difficulty looking up and down without bending the neck. Slowing of thinking/processing and executive problems similar to those in *corticobasal degeneration* are reflective of the subcortical damage in progressive supranuclear palsy.

Those with another protein, FUS, present, but no tau
These abnormal protein complexes may occur in numerous parts of the brain, and the symptoms are consequently quite varied.

Those with no tau or FUS, but with other abnormal proteins present (ubiquitin and TDP-43)
There are multiple subtypes, but this group has an association with the clinical syndrome of semantic dementia, a type of language variant frontotemporal dementia mentioned earlier.

Neuroimaging in frontotemporal dementia
Although both functional and structural brain scans of someone with frontotemporal dementia may be normal early in the disease process, there are characteristic features that help identify it as the condition progresses. MRI scans may show shrinkage (atrophy) of the frontal or temporal lobes, and functional scans (such as PET, SPECT and fMRI scans) may show reduced activity in these same areas.

Progression of frontotemporal dementia
Frontotemporal dementia tends to develop gradually. It also develops at an earlier age than Alzheimer's disease – typically in the

sixth or seventh decade of life. This can lead to specific challenges, as the affected individual may develop dementia at a point when they are otherwise physically robust and healthy. This means that behavioural changes, including aggression and agitation, which are often pronounced in frontotemporal dementia, can be considerably more problematic for those caring for the individual experiencing the disease. Complicating matters, its earlier age of onset means that the person with frontotemporal dementia is commonly still working, and there can be significant occupational fallout before the disease is picked up.

The mean duration of lifespan from diagnosis to death is five to eight years; a shorter lifespan is expected with the behavioural variant compared with the language variants. Over this time, there will generally be progressive impairment, though this can sometimes proceed quite slowly. There can be considerable variability to the prognosis.

Some presentations of behavioural variant frontotemporal dementia show little or no decline over many years. These are known as *frontotemporal dementia phenocopies*. These are very much the exception rather than the rule, however, and the vast majority of frontotemporal dementia patients do decline noticeably with time.

Alcohol-related dementia

When taken in moderation, alcohol can have beneficial social side effects. Unfortunately, however, there is no escaping the fact that alcohol is a poison, and when drunk in excess of recommended amounts, and especially for an enduring period, it can cause numerous health problems. These include liver disease, high blood pressure and heart failure, certain cancers (especially of the digestive tract) and mental health disorders, such as depression and anxiety.

Alcohol can also have a detrimental effect on cognitive function, both in the acute state of intoxication and if taken excessively over a long period. In this latter scenario, cognitive impairment may persist even when a person has been sober for some time, and may even become permanent.

Is a little better than none?

The amount of alcohol in a drink is usually measured in terms of grams of ethanol. This is a product of the percentage alcohol in the drink multiplied by the volume of the drink. Ten grams of ethanol equals one standard drink, or standard unit. In Australia, producers of alcoholic drinks are required by law to inform the buyer how many standard units a drink contains. This should be listed directly on the can or the label of beer, wine or spirits.

For the general population, there is considerable variability in the advice given about alcohol consumption. Many experts believe there is no safe level of drinking – that each drink increases the risk of some adverse short-term or long-term health outcome. For this reason, certain organisations – including the World Health Organization – feel it is best not to provide specific advice about how much to drink. In Australia, the National Health and Medical Research Council has recently published draft guidelines that incorporate this thinking – that the less you choose to drink, the lower your risk of alcohol-related harm – but it does provide quantitative advice for healthy men and women: not to drink more than ten units per week, and four units in any one day.

There seems to be a significant difference in individual vulnerability to the effects of alcohol: some people appear to be able to consume relatively large quantities over a long period of time and have no clinically significant impairment of cognition, while others who have drunk considerably less may have much more obvious sequelae (or health conditions). It is difficult to predict who is likely to fall into which category.

It remains unclear whether low to moderate levels of alcohol consumption are protective against some forms of dementia, including vascular dementia and Alzheimer's disease. Alcohol has a theoretical antioxidant effect, which could be of some benefit, and its moderate use may confer some heart and vascular benefits. Some studies have shown that individuals who consume moderate levels of alcohol (between 1 and 14 standard units per week) have lower rates of dementia. The 'non-drinkers' in the studies may have included people who had previously drunk heavily but who had given up by the time of the study, however. Their risk of developing dementia may therefore have been elevated by this previous excessive consumption but falsely attributed to lifelong teetotalism.

Another study demonstrated that binge drinking in midlife (defined as drinking the equivalent of one bottle of wine in one sitting at least monthly) was associated with an increased risk of dementia later in life. This raises the question of how the pattern of alcohol consumption, rather than absolute quantities drunk, may influence risk. Again, this remains unsatisfactorily answered.

Another unanswered question is whether one type of alcohol (red wine, white wine, beer or spirits) might be better than another when it comes to brain health. Many studies have not differentiated between different types of alcohol, though some have seemed to suggest a specific benefit for red wine, which has a number of antioxidants that may stave off oxidative stress and chronic inflammation. One of these antioxidants, a polyphenol called resveratrol, has garnered particular attention as it seems to have cardioprotective effects, and in mice at least has been shown to reduce beta-amyloid in the brain. More recently, however, there have been a number of studies suggesting there is also benefit to be had from drinking less than heavy amounts of beer. More research is clearly needed to decipher where the truth lies, and how much of what we do is wishful drinking!

Brain damage caused by alcohol

What is clear is that chronic excessive use of alcohol is likely to cause damage to the brain. Alcohol-related dementia (ARD) falls under the broader category of alcohol-related cognitive impairment. The other recognised syndrome in this category is *Wernicke-Korsakoff syndrome*, also known as *alcohol-induced persisting amnestic syndrome*.

Wernicke-Korsakoff syndrome

This comprises two conditions that often occur together, or in short sequence: *Wernicke encephalopathy* and *Korsakoff syndrome*. They are considered to be related to a lack of vitamin B1 (thiamine), something that is very common in those who use alcohol excessively. B1 deficiency can also occur in those with a chronic illness or after weight-loss surgery.

Wernicke encephalopathy is an acute state of altered mental function, classically characterised by confusion, loss of muscle coordination (ataxia) and visual changes (especially a condition called nystagmus, but also double vision and drooping of the eyelids).

Korsakoff syndrome tends to develop as Wernicke encephalopathy symptoms start to resolve. It probably develops as a consequence of damage to limbic structures, specifically the thalamus and part of the hypothalamus known as the *mamillary bodies*. These latter structures are closely connected to the hippocampus, accounting for one of the chief symptoms: an inability to form new memories. The loss of memory in those experiencing this condition can be severe.

Korsakoff syndrome may also present with a phenomenon known as *confabulation*, which denotes the creation of false memories in the absence of any intent to deceive, and that the person believes to be true. This is also known as 'honest lying'; it can be seen as a way of 'filling in the gaps' of a story that has been forgotten.

Alcohol-related dementia (ARD)

Excessive and prolonged alcohol use can lead to permanent damage to the structure and function of the brain. Research demonstrates that males who consume more than six and women who consume more than four standard alcoholic drinks per day, over an extended period (years), seem to be at increased risk of developing alcohol-related dementia. The precise quantity required to cause ARD is subject to debate, however.

A number of mechanisms have been proposed to explain the damaging effect of alcohol on the brain. These include:

- *The 'neurotoxicity' hypothesis.* This suggests nerve cells are damaged through oxidative stress (see Chapter 8), the toxic effects of a neurotransmitter called glutamate and the impaired formation of new nerve cells.
- *Disruption of the cholinergic system*, especially in the basal forebrain (the part at the bottom front of the brain). This would account for the noted problems in attention, learning and memory.

- *Vitamin B1 (thiamine) deficiency.* In a similar way to Wernicke-Korsakoff syndrome, lack of this vitamin may cause the less-reversible syndrome of ARD.

Whatever the exact cause, the brains of those with ARD show a number of abnormalities, including loss of white matter (especially in the prefrontal cortex, corpus callosum and cerebellum), and changes to the structure of nerve cells, again in the frontal areas and cerebellum. The frontal areas show shrinkage and decreased activity on brain scans. The alterations in the structure of the nerve cells seem to inhibit their ability to communicate with each other. It is unclear whether the nerve cells actually die, but alcohol does seem to inhibit the growth of new nerve cells – something that otherwise is a lifelong process.

Long-term alcohol abuse also appears to be associated with loss of volume of the hippocampi – potentially the cause of specific problems with learning new information. It is not confirmed, however, that alcohol causes this shrinking, as it may be that the hippocampi of alcoholics were small prior to the alcohol abuse, which might even contribute to the risk of developing problems with alcohol in the first place.

Signs and symptoms of ARD

Studies suggest that ARD occurs at a younger age than other dementias, and that it's more common in males and in those who are socially isolated.

The distribution of the damage in the brain tends to explain the common symptoms and signs. In thinking about this, it can be helpful to consider how people act when they are drunk, because there are similarities with the changes seen in ARD. The preferential effect on the frontal lobe may result in certain behavioural changes, such as disinhibition and poor impulse control, socially inappropriate behaviours, apathy, aggression and a disregard for the effects of one's behaviours on others.

From a cognitive perspective, tasks that involve planning, organisation and judgement are often particularly poorly performed – these are all executive functions dependent on the frontal lobe. Working memory and attention may be impaired, as may visuospatial skills and motor speed. Language skills are typically well preserved – individuals can speak well, giving a false impression in general conversation, though on formal cognitive testing there are obvious problems. ARD is considered to have both cortical and subcortical elements, something backed up by at least one study looking at SPECT scans (see Chapter 13), which show the level of activity in the brain to be lower in certain parts of both areas.

As with Alzheimer's disease, memory complaints appear to relate initially to short-term memory. Individuals may struggle to learn new information or focus on a conversation. Recent events are poorly remembered. With more severe illness, there is also a loss of long-term memory. Individuals may make errors when recalling remote information. This sometimes manifests as confabulation, mentioned earlier.

Psychiatric symptoms may also accompany ARD, with an increased risk of depression, anxiety, personality changes and psychosis.

Progression of ARD

One unique and positive aspect of ARD is that it is not as inexorably progressive as some other forms of dementia. Stopping drinking can halt further progression; indeed, it is reasonable to anticipate a degree of recovery with enduring abstinence from alcohol. The degree and nature of any recovery seems to be mediated by the duration of abstinence more than by the absolute lifetime alcohol use. Older drinkers may show less recovery, and risk factors for other dementias also influence the outcome.

Subcortical dementias

As we saw in Chapter 1, the brain can be considered as having both cortical and subcortical elements. When we see the brain from the outside, it is really the cortex we are seeing – the outer layer of the brain, with its characteristic twists, turns and grooved channels. Below this wrapping layer, there are numerous structures that are collectively known as the subcortex. The purpose of the subcortical elements is quite different to that of their cortical counterparts.

The subcortical structures include the limbic system, the basal ganglia and the cerebellum. Symptoms associated with damage to this region differ from those arising from a damaged cortex.

Although there is some controversy as to the value of distinguishing dementias on the basis of this difference in location, it is helpful to consider that dementia may be primarily cortical or subcortical in nature, or a mix, as the following table sets out.

Dementia	Subcortical	Cortical	Mixed
Parkinson's disease	x		
Alzheimer's disease		x	
Dementia with Lewy bodies			x
Vascular dementia	x	x	x
Huntington's disease	x		
Frontotemporal dementia		x	x
HIV-related dementia	x		
Creutzfeldt-Jakob disease			x

Predominant pattern of disease in early forms of different dementias.

There may also be a change in the distribution of the underlying brain tissue damage in different dementias as they progress, meaning that what was once a typical cortical dementia may also develop a subcortical component (or vice versa).

Symptoms and signs of subcortical dementias

Typically, individuals with subcortical dementias tend to have more early disturbance of movement (e.g. due to parkinsonism) and more early neuropsychiatric symptoms (such as depression or apathy) than those with cortical dementia.

There may be more noticeable reduction in processing speed (the ability to think and respond to what is occurring in the environment), mirrored by slowing of thoughts in general (*bradyphrenia*) and of movements (*bradykinesia*). Given time, however, individuals with subcortical dementias often respond appropriately and accurately, suggesting the problem may be one of disordered retrieval rather than acquisition. Cueing is often of benefit in helping individuals remember. Language function often tends to be normal, though there may be abnormalities of speech, such as a soft voice (*hypophonia*) or slurring (*dysarthria*). Executive function is also often affected, something that may be related to poor connectivity between subcortical areas and the frontal lobe.

It should be pointed out that being told you have a subcortical dementia, just like being told you have dementia more generally, does not give you a specific diagnosis. Let's now consider a few specific causes of subcortical and mixed dementia.

Huntington's disease

Also known as *Huntington's chorea*, this a condition that, in the large majority of cases, is inherited from a parent (though 10 per cent are related to a new gene mutation). A child of an affected parent has a 50 per cent chance of inheriting the disease. It arises from the mutation of a certain protein (huntingtin) that is toxic to certain cells, including those in the brain. The *striatum* – a part of the basal ganglia – is affected early, influencing movement and motivation.

Although it is a rare condition, Huntington's disease can be particularly troublesome and distressing as it usually develops early – normally between the ages of 30 and 50 – and affects otherwise healthy individuals.

Cognitive deficits typically occur later in the disease, and the first signs and symptoms can be non-specific – subtle changes in mood, for example. After a time, *choreiform* movements develop. These are distinctive jerky, involuntary body movements that can become quite dramatic – sometimes with unintended violent flinging movements of the limbs. Physical capabilities deteriorate, and speaking, swallowing and chewing can become difficult. Eventually, the ability to walk vanishes. Unfortunately, individuals with Huntington's disease often lose insight into the extent of their problems.

The cognitive deficits in Huntington's disease include pronounced executive dysfunction (such as poor planning, abstraction and inhibition). Memory deficits develop as the disease progresses, and include problems in working memory, short-term memory and long-term memory. Even procedural memory (overlearned memory) tends to be affected. The disease also has a fairly high burden of neuropsychiatric features, including depression, anxiety, irritability, apathy, aggression and obsessive–compulsive symptoms.

Both MRI brain scans and PET scans may show characteristic patterns in those with Huntington's disease, though it is important to confirm a diagnosis with genetic testing, particularly owing to the need to identify the risk to other family members.

Parkinson's disease

The classic triad of Parkinson's disease involves rigidity/stiffness (of muscles), bradykinesia (slowing of movement) and a tremor (most noticeable in the hands, classically described as a 'pill rolling tremor'). An individual with this condition often has a shuffling gait and appears hesitant when starting movement. They may also stoop forward, and their face may show little expression. Their writing often becomes small (*micrographia*) and their voice soft and muffled (*hypophonia*).

Parkinson's disease was once considered to be purely a disease of motor (movement) function – understandably, given these are the most obvious signs. It is now recognised as a condition that affects multiple bodily systems, such as those involving cognitive and psychological domains, as well as those governing basic aspects of the nervous system, like temperature regulation and blood pressure.

The damage to the brain in Parkinson's disease is caused by the abnormal deposition of a protein known as *alpha synuclein* (also known as Lewy bodies after their discoverer, a neurologist named Frederic Lewy). This protein tends to accumulate within nerve cells in various subcortical structures, including the basal ganglia, hence the presence of movement problems. Much of the classic presentation of Parkinson's disease is due to the loss of dopaminergic neurons, associated with a lack of *dopamine*, a type of neurotransmitter (like acetylcholine).

Cognitive impairment in Parkinson's disease is very common, though associated dementia usually occurs in the later stages of the disease (on average, ten years after onset). Between 50 and 80 per cent of individuals with Parkinson's disease ultimately experience dementia – referred to as *Parkinson's disease dementia.*

Consistent with the subcortical pathology, cognitive problems tend to be most prominently executive dysfunction, difficulties with attention and concentration, and problems with learning new skills. With progression of the disease, short-term memory deteriorates, as does word-finding ability. Visuospatial skills also tend to be affected, and individuals may have difficulty judging distances.

Neuropsychiatric features may also accompany Parkinson's disease, along with the associated dementia. Psychotic symptoms (hallucinations and delusions) and mood changes (depression) may arise, as may irritability and anxiety. Specific sleep difficulties are sometimes noticeable – for example, *rapid eye movement* (REM) *sleep behaviour disorder* (RBD). Since dreaming occurs in the REM phase of sleep, this may cause an individual to 'act out' their dreams, including by thrashing about violently or screaming and shouting. This is discussed in more detail in Chapter 17.

Structural brain scans such as MRIs and CT scans are generally unhelpful to those with Parkinson's disease, except to exclude other causes (some types of vascular disease may cause symptoms resembling Parkinson's disease, for example). PET scans may show low levels of dopamine in the brain, though these are not routinely used in diagnosis of the condition. Parkinson's disease thus remains a largely clinical diagnosis – one that relies on detecting certain signs and symptoms rather than tests.

Dementia with Lewy bodies

There is considerable pathological and clinical overlap between Parkinson's disease and dementia with Lewy bodies. As the name suggests, Lewy bodies also underpin the problems in this condition, and in fact *Lewy body disease* is an umbrella term that includes both dementia with Lewy bodies and Parkinson's disease dementia. The distinguishing factor between the two conditions is the sequence of symptoms: in Parkinson's disease dementia the movement disorder comes first, while in dementia with Lewy bodies the cognitive symptoms come first.

Dementia with Lewy bodies is actually both a cortical and subcortical dementia; the Lewy bodies are spread throughout the cerebral cortex and hippocampus, and also the midbrain and brainstem. The brain in Lewy body disease demonstrates cortical and subcortical atrophy (shrinkage), including of the temporal, frontal and parietal lobes. Loss of volume can also be seen in the hippocampus, amygdala and basal ganglia. Acetylcholine is depleted, possibly to an even greater degree than seen in Alzheimer's disease, and dopamine levels are also affected, which accounts for the movement disorder that often accompanies the condition.

Dementia with Lewy bodies is considered by some to be the second-most common cause of late-onset dementia, possibly accounting for 20 per cent of cases, though this is not without controversy. Men seem to be more at risk than women. Like Alzheimer's disease, age appears to be the biggest risk factor for developing the condition, and in a similar fashion the underlying pathology (plaques and tangles in Alzheimer's, and Lewy bodies in dementia with Lewy bodies) can also be found in the brains of healthy individuals. Little is known about other risk factors, though having Parkinson's disease results in an increased chance of acquiring the disease. Genetics do not seem to play a major role in risk generation. There is also an apparent link between Alzheimer's disease and Lewy body disease, with Lewy bodies not uncommonly being found in the brains of those with Alzheimer's disease.

Lewy body dementia is often misdiagnosed as delirium, a condition with which it shares some features. One of the early signs of dementia with Lewy bodies may be REM sleep behaviour disorder, mentioned earlier.

The symptoms and signs of dementia with Lewy bodies are often quite distinctive, and include:

- *Visual hallucinations.* These are experienced by 80 per cent of those affected, and can be very detailed. Typically, the hallucinations are of adults, children or animals.
- Prominent difficulties with *visuospatial tasks.*
- *Executive difficulties* and *attentional problems.*

- Motor features of Parkinson's disease (*tremor, rigidity* and *bradykinesia*). These tend to be less severe than seen in Parkinson's disease dementia, at least initially.
- Marked fluctuation in *cognitive abilities* and *level of alertness*. Individuals may appear relatively lucid and alert one moment, and then quickly become drowsy and confused. This may happen multiple times in one day.
- *Autonomic dysfunction.* The autonomic system is part of our nervous system and regulates, among other things, our blood pressure, pulse rate and temperature. Patients with dementia with Lewy bodies may have marked variations in these parameters: they may experience a significant drop in blood pressure, for example, when moving from a sitting position to standing (*postural hypotension*).
- *Neuroleptic sensitivity.* When patients with dementia with Lewy bodies are given certain medications (antipsychotics such as risperidone for agitation, for example) they can react very badly, developing suddenly worsening sedation, cognition and possibly irreversible parkinsonism.

There is a great deal of variability in the prognosis with dementia with Lewy bodies, though it is a progressive condition. The average duration of the disease is five to seven years.

AIDS dementia complex (ADC)

Acquired immune deficiency syndrome (AIDS) is an illness caused by the human immunodeficiency virus (HIV), which affects multiple systems in the body. It first came to public attention in the 1980s. At that stage there were very few treatments available and it was considered a terminal disease, though over the intervening decades there has been much progress and it is probably now better conceived of as a chronic and manageable disease like rheumatoid arthritis or diabetes.

The dementia that can arise with AIDS is not common, especially in the early stages of the disease, but it can occur in up to 7 per cent of individuals not receiving antiviral medication. The virus indirectly affects nerve cells and thus causes damage to the brain.

The symptoms are again consistent with a subcortical process: difficulties with concentration, slowing of thinking, mood changes and problems with gait and movement. Later, executive problems become more pronounced, apathy may occur, and continence of bowel and bladder may be lost.

The diagnosis of ADC is a clinical one, usually made by examination of a patient known to have HIV, including cognitive examination. Cerebrospinal fluid can be taken and assessed for the presence of HIV. Other tests (including blood tests and brain scans) may be performed to exclude other causes of cognitive impairment.

Use of antiretroviral drugs can prevent and treat ADC, though the treatment is often not terribly effective once the damage has been done. Medications can also be used to treat the sequelae of ADC, including psychiatric symptoms.

Hydrocephalus

This condition, literally meaning 'water in the brain', is the result of an abnormal build-up of cerebrospinal fluid in the ventricles in the brain. These structures may not be strictly subcortical, though ventricular enlargement causes, via pressure on the brain tissue, a dementia that is typically subcortical in nature. Hydrocephalus is associated with a classic 'triad' of symptoms – walking difficulties (gait disturbance), dementia and poor bladder control (urinary incontinence) – though not everyone has all three symptoms. Gait disturbance is usually the earliest feature. Movement appears to be slowed, and the individual may walk with a broad-based gait – that is, with the feet kept further apart than usual, for greater stability. The gait may also be shuffling in nature.

Although most cases occur for unknown reasons, hydrocephalus can occur as a consequence of another problem, such as a brain tumour, infection, head injury or inflammation.

The cognitive symptoms of hydrocephalus reflect subcortical damage and often include poor attention, slowed thinking (bradyphrenia) and forgetfulness. Language problems are not common.

Brain scans can be particularly helpful in identifying hydrocephalus because they reveal the enlargement of the ventricles and a flattening of other brain structures.

Use of more specialised techniques, most notably studies of cerebrospinal fluid flow, can help confirm the diagnosis in those with equivocal findings on other brain scans.

Treatment of hydrocephalus is essentially surgical, with a shunt (tube) being placed such that one end is in the ventricles and the other is in the abdominal cavity; this allows drainage of the cerebrospinal fluid, relieving pressure in the ventricles. Although shunting can result in significant improvement in some symptoms, this is more the case when the disease is caught early. Unfortunately, once a dementia is manifest, there may be limited improvement in cognition even when the cerebrospinal fluid is drained.

Hydrocephalus also quite commonly occurs alongside other dementias, including Alzheimer's disease and vascular dementia.

★

This marks the end of Part One, in which we've discussed the healthy brain, what we can do to keep it that way and the uncertain role of supplements. We have also looked at the effects of ageing on the brain, as well as syndromes that represent something more than ageing but fall short of being dementia. Finally, we have talked about reversible causes of cognitive impairment, as well as the commoner types of dementia and how they present.

In Part Two, our focus will shift to the lived experience of dementia. First we'll look at how cognitive impairment is assessed – who is involved and what they do – and what to expect with the progression of various types of dementia. As we have touched on, those with dementia may experience not only problems with thinking, but also physical, psychological and behavioural challenges, and we will discuss how best to manage these. Importantly, we'll explore the pivotal and often difficult role of carers, and consider how to manage the burden of care. Part Two also provides advice on legal and ethical issues, end-of-life care and how to navigate the somewhat complex aged-care system.

Living with Dementia

SECTION I
Being Assessed for Dementia

10

The Assessment Process

- It is best for dementia to be picked up early.

- Determining whether someone has dementia often involves numerous health professionals. These individuals may also help manage dementia as it progresses.

- Health professionals play different, but partly overlapping roles, assessing areas such as physical health, cognition, daily functioning and social supports.

- Memory clinics often exist in larger metropolitan hospitals. These have the advantage of bringing many health professionals together in a multidisciplinary team to discuss an individual's problems.

It's not uncommon for me to see individuals who have had symptoms of dementia for many years, and who by the time I assess them are in the more severe stages of the illness. This is sometimes due to the patient's or carer's belief that there's no point finding out if they have dementia as nothing can be done about it anyway. This is incorrect; as we shall see, there are a number of interventions that can be very helpful for the individual experiencing dementia, as well as for their carers.

It is always best to try to confirm the presence of dementia early. There are numerous reasons for this:

- First, the medications we use to treat certain types of dementia are much more beneficial when the disease is mild. The same is probably true of lifestyle interventions.
- Second, an early diagnosis allows individuals and their families to *plan* for the future, before they become incapable of making relevant legal and lifestyle decisions.
- Third, although being told you have dementia can be harrowing, knowing there is a cause for your symptoms can be in some ways comforting.
- Finally, becoming more knowledgeable about the behavioural and psychological symptoms associated with dementia – which, if they manifest, can cause great disruption to personal and intimate relationships – can mitigate against personal damage. Knowing that a difficult behaviour is not deliberate can make it a lot easier to deal with.

Broadly, there are four steps in the process of medically assessing someone who has presented with cognitive problems:

- Taking the patient's medical history
- Conducting a physical examination
- Testing their memory and other cognitive abilities
- Organising medical investigations such as blood tests, urine tests and imaging of the brain.

These elements of assessment will be discussed in some detail over the next few chapters, but let's first look at who may be involved in the process. There can be a number of health professionals who ideally work together when assessing someone with cognitive impairment. Many of them may stay involved beyond a diagnosis to manage the various issues that arise.

General practitioners (GPs)

Unless cognitive problems are discovered by specialists looking after an individual when they are in hospital (or possibly in an outpatients' clinic), the GP is usually the medical professional who starts the process of assessment. This is appropriate, as they're often the one who knows the patient best and can therefore judge whether there has been the change in functioning and cognition that is the prerequisite of dementia. The GP may take a history (that is, ask questions about what has happened), perform some basic cognitive testing and organise the routine blood and urine tests that are performed as part of the 'work-up'. Sometimes the GP is confident enough to diagnose the type of dementia themselves, but often they seek the help of specialists before confirming this.

Specialist doctors

Three types of medical specialist commonly assess people with memory loss. These are *neurologists, psychogeriatricians* and *geriatricians*. All three have obtained a medical degree and then specialised in their particular area.

Neurologists

As the name suggests, neurologists specialise in problems to do with the nervous system. This includes the brain, and therefore dementia. They may see patients of any age, though in the context of cognitive problems, they are often asked to see a patient who is younger, or for whom there is suspicion of a less common form of dementia such as those caused by viruses, multiple sclerosis or disease processes affecting the subcortex, including Parkinson's disease and Huntington's disease. Neurologists may have ready access to specific neurological tests that are utilised in rarer dementias, such as lumbar punctures and electroencephalography (EEGs, which test electrical activity in the brain).

Psychogeriatricians

These practitioners (of whom I am one) specialise first in psychiatry, and then old-age psychiatry. They are often asked to consult on older patients, including those for whom a commoner form of dementia is considered likely (Alzheimer's disease, vascular dementia, dementia with Lewy bodies, frontotemporal dementia and so on). They are also frequently involved when there are prominent psychological or behavioural changes, or where there is uncertainty about whether a psychological problem (such as depression) may be causing the cognitive impairment.

Geriatricians

Specialising in medicine in the elderly, these doctors have considerable overlap with psychogeriatricians, though they are particularly skilled at managing physical health conditions that occur with ageing and that may be contributing to, or complicating, cognitive decline. They commonly see the more usual types of late-onset dementia such as Alzheimer's disease, vascular dementia and dementia with Lewy bodies.

Allied health professionals

Allied health professionals are those who work in the area of health but who are not doctors, nurses or dentists. Individuals who work in allied health include psychologists and neuropsychologists, occupational therapists, physiotherapists, social workers, speech therapists and dieticians. They have generally completed tertiary qualifications in their chosen field, and often play a crucial role both in the assessment of someone with possible dementia and in their ongoing care.

Psychologists and counsellors

Psychologists may become involved if there is a prominent psychological component to the cognitive syndrome. They are tertiary-educated in their chosen field, undertaking at least a degree in psychology. They can provide therapy for those experiencing dementia (especially early in the disease), as well as for their carers. Importantly, they can help with the process of psychological adjustment to the diagnosis. Counsellors can also be very helpful in providing emotional support to those diagnosed with a form of dementia, as well as to their carers.

Neuropsychologists

These are psychologists who have undertaken specific further training in cognitive assessment. They can be invaluable when, after the usual cognitive testing and investigations, the diagnosis remains uncertain.

Occupational therapists (OTs)

These specialists can be very helpful in the initial review of a patient with possible dementia by performing *functional assessments*. As we saw in Part One, for dementia to be considered likely there has to be some impairment of function as a consequence of the cognitive problems. Sometimes it is not enough to simply ask an individual or their carer about their functional limitations, and a practical test is required.

In those experiencing mild difficulties, tests may involve money management or cooking skills, for instance; in those with more advanced impairment, the focus may be on toileting, dressing and bathing. In some cases OTs also perform driving tests, and they can advise on equipment that might improve the safety or comfort of an individual's home environment (such as stair rails or a shower chair).

Physiotherapists

Physiotherapists specialise in assessing and optimising the musculoskeletal system, including looking at balance and muscle strength. Ageing alone can cause disturbances in these areas, and they can be exacerbated in dementia. Falls are of particular concern, and physiotherapists can help individuals improve their strength in relevant muscle groups in order to reduce the risk. They may do this through guided exercises or balance training, and can advise on the need for mobility aids such as wheelie walkers. Physiotherapists can also suggest and apply strategies to manage musculoskeletal pain, such as massage or stretching.

Social workers

Professionals trained in this discipline are adept at investigating and optimising the social dimensions of dementia. This may involve looking at accommodation circumstances, family or other supports, and associated risks. A social worker may also consider an individual's financial situation, and ensure they have access to adequate professional support. Informally, social workers can be immensely helpful in providing emotional and psychological support during the diagnostic process and beyond.

Speech therapists

The two main roles of a speech therapist in dementia are to assess swallowing abilities and to assess and manage communication problems. The reflex to swallow may become impaired as a consequence of dementia, and this leads to a potential risk of aspiration (taking food or fluid into the lungs) and chest infection. Speech therapists advise on the integrity of the swallow reflex and whether a patient should limit certain types of food or fluid. Difficulty communicating is a very common accompaniment of dementia, and speech therapists can evaluate language function and advise on ways in which communication can be optimised.

Dieticians

Although dieticians are not commonly involved in the initial diagnostic assessment, they advise on the type and quantity of food and fluid that individuals may need. They may become involved when there is concern about undernutrition (by looking at the use of supplements or variations to diet, for example) or obesity.

Nurses

Nurses, being responsible for managing day-to-day medical concerns and helping with medication management, are often involved both in an initial dementia assessment and in the ongoing management of those with the condition. They may provide care for an individual at home or in an aged-care facility, administer medications and attend to physical health concerns such as ulcers. They may be the first to flag cognitive and functional problems. Nurses also provide much-needed practical and emotional support to carers and their relatives.

Formal care providers

This term refers to those providing help at home or assisting individuals in residential care. Their role may include helping someone with showering, helping them dress and supervising meals. Often, these are the people who know the individual best and can identify changes that may suggest the development of dementia. They can provide important information about someone's day-to-day functioning, as well as how best to approach care and what sort of risks may be present.

Memory clinics

Although I currently work exclusively in private practice with individuals referred to me by their GPs, I have had the privilege of working in a number of *memory clinics*, both in Australia and the United Kingdom. These clinics, usually run through the public health system, are, in my opinion, the optimal way to be assessed, as they are usually run by a multidisciplinary team that includes a number of the professionals described above. An individual presenting with memory loss can therefore be comprehensively assessed and discussed by the members of the team.

11

Medical History

- The first step in determining whether someone has dementia is to take a detailed history of the problem.

- Having an informant or carer at the assessment is important, as the patient may not have insight into the extent of their problems.

- Psychological and physical conditions can mimic dementia and need to be enquired about. Likewise, medications can cause cognitive problems and should be assessed.

- Our personal history can have a significant effect on how dementia presents and how we cope with it.

- Assessing risk (to oneself and to others) is an important aspect of history gathering.

- Knowing who will be responsible for health and other decisions as the dementia progresses is important to establish early on.

When doctors ask questions to try to establish a diagnosis, or at least narrow it down to a small number of possibilities (a *differential*), it is called *taking a history*.

It is important first to get a general sense of the person's circumstances. Some of this is termed the *social history*. Regardless of the nature and extent of their difficulties, this is extremely relevant and may influence what approach is taken after a diagnosis is made.

Examples of these initial questions may include:

- 'Why do you think you are coming to this consultation?' This immediately casts light on the extent of *insight* (awareness) they may have about their problems.
- 'Do you live alone?' Someone in this position is clearly more at risk.
- 'Are you married? Do you have someone who can help you at home, or who you look after? How is their health?' Knowing the health status of a dependent or carer is important when clarifying the need for supports and potential risk issues.
- 'What is the physical layout of your home?' This may identify specific risks, such as the presence of a large number of stairs or a gas cooker.
- 'What supports do you have? Do you have family, friends or health professionals who help you?' This may dictate how much needs to be done immediately and into the future.
- 'What is/was your occupation?' This may give a clue into the patient's *premorbid* (before the problems began) intellectual functioning. This is important in determining whether there has been a change in function, which is a key aspect of the condition.
- 'Have you appointed a substitute decision-maker? Has a plan been enacted?' This clarifies who may be making important decisions for the patient into the future.

The next step in determining whether a dementia may be present is to evaluate whether there is evidence of cognitive impairment, and whether this represents a change from a previous situation.

As the individual experiencing cognitive impairment may have limited insight into the extent of their problems, it is very important to gather collateral information. This involves speaking with someone who (preferably) knows the patient well and has known them since before the onset of problems. Usually this is a spouse or other family member. Sometimes this can be a delicate issue, as the carer may not want to be honest in front of the patient, lest they be seen as critical or challenging, though I emphasise the need to gather as much information as possible so that the condition can be recognised and, if appropriate, treated early.

Sometimes at this early stage I will use a formal scale such as the Informant Questionnaire on Cognitive Decline in the Elderly (IQCODE). This is a brief questionnaire (available as a PDF online) given to the carer. Its questions aim to identify whether there has been a deterioration in specific areas compared with ten years before. These may include financial management, misplacing objects and forgetting recent events. This at least generates a conversation about potential issues.

Early in the evaluation, I also try to get a sense of the time frame of the symptoms. As we have seen, most types of dementia present with a gradual onset of symptoms, occurring over months or years. There are exceptions, such as single-infarct dementia, but this is the general rule.

- If the onset is *acute* (in the space of hours to days), delirium is much more likely. This is also known as an *acute confusional state* and can have many causes (see Chapter 5).
- If it is *subacute* (weeks to months), the possibility of a psychological cause such as depression should be considered (see Chapter 5).

As we saw in Part One, the specific symptoms and signs of dementia depend on the underlying cause, and memory loss may not be the most prominent issue. When individuals are referred to me by their GP, I usually have some indication of the presenting problem – whether memory loss is the main concern, for instance, or whether a change in behaviour or language has been observed, or other symptoms.

Although I may place different emphasis on particular questions depending on an individual's symptoms, there are a number of areas that I always enquire about. These include cognitive changes such as memory function, orientation, executive function, language and praxis, psychological function, problems with physical health, and medications. Family history may also be important, as may substance use. Let's now look at what questions can be asked to clarify these different areas.

Cognitive function

See Chapter 1 for a detailed description of these functions.

Memory function

I try to clarify whether the deficit in memory relates to short-term memory or long-term memory. It is usually the former, probably because newer memories have not been stored as effectively as older ones.

Questions with which I assess the presence of short-term memory loss include:

- Has the patient forgotten details of recent conversations?
- Have they been repetitive in their conversations?
- Have there been frequent episodes of misplacing objects and not being able to find them?
- Have they frequently forgotten why they have entered a room?
- Have they struggled to remember to take their medications, or to remember important events or appointments?
- Have bills been left unpaid?
- Have they struggled to remember new information or work out how to use new devices such as phones?

It is not uncommon for the person experiencing dementia to have poor insight into their problems, or to want to minimise them. It is therefore very important to ask someone who spends time with the person, or knows them well, what their opinion is about the above questions.

I also try to establish whether cueing is helpful – does giving a hint about what has been forgotten jog their memory? This can indicate that vascular disease may be part of the problem, or that a psychological factor such as depression or anxiety is present. Cueing tends to be less helpful in Alzheimer's disease, where the information has simply not 'gone in' in the first place.

Long-term memory deficits can be identified by asking whether the individual remembers important events from months or years ago. Corroboration by someone who has experienced these same events is obviously important. Such deficits are not common in most early dementias, though often occur as the dementia progresses.

Orientation
This is closely related to short-term memory function and involves an awareness of where one is, both in space and in time. Questions I use to assess this include:

- Has the patient become lost in familiar surroundings, such as while driving or at a shopping centre?
- Have they ever wandered away from their home and become disoriented? Has this occurred at night? This may also give an indication of the risks posed by the problem.

Executive skills and frontal-lobe function
- Has the person struggled with cooking? Paying bills?
- Have they been absentminded or had trouble paying attention? This may indicate a problem with working memory. This may be especially noticeable in environments where there are multiple stimuli, such as lots of people or extraneous noise.
- Have they been easily distracted?
- Have they been more impulsive than usual (acting without thinking)?
- Have they had difficulty with planning meals, events, holidays and so on?
- Have they had difficulty controlling their emotions?
- Have they been uncharacteristically irritable? Frustrated? Apathetic (that is, showing a loss of 'get up and go')?
- Have they struggled moving from one task to another, or become fixated on certain topics?
- Has there been a deterioration in their social behaviour? Do they seem disinhibited or uncharacteristically rude?
- Have they made inappropriate sexual remarks?
- Do they seem not to care about the impact of their behaviours on others?
- Have there been any changes in dietary preference, especially a hankering for sweet foods?

- Have they seemed less flexible?
- Have they become emotionally aloof?
- Has there been a change in their personality?

Again, asking these same questions of someone who knows the patient well can reveal problems that otherwise may be denied and remain hidden.

Language function
- Does the individual sometimes struggle to find the right word in a conversation? *Expressive dysphasia* is a phenomenon usually associated with damage to part of the frontal lobe (Broca's area); it is classically seen as a consequence of stroke, though is not uncommon with dementia.
- Do they seem not to understand what is being asked of them or to follow simple commands? This may suggest *receptive dysphasia*, a problem with understanding the spoken word rather than expressing it, and is often caused by damage to part of the temporal lobe (Wernicke's area).
- Has the patient's speech become vaguer? Do they tend to talk around the point (circumlocution) because they cannot remember the right word to use?
- Have there been word substitutions?

Praxis
- Does the subject struggle with coordination?
- Do they find it difficult to manipulate objects that should be familiar to them? Can they put their clothes on correctly? Brush their hair? Shower themselves?

Visuospatial skills, including gnosis
- Has the patient struggled with judging distances or had problems with depth perception? This may result in falls or difficulties negotiating uneven surfaces or stairs. Even sitting, including using the toilet, can become difficult as they may misjudge where the seat is.
- Has there been evidence of impaired recognition of familiar

objects, people or colours?
- Have they failed to recognise the details of the environment they are in?
- Has reading or writing become a problem?

Calculation
- Has the patient struggled with using money, counting out change or performing sums?

Psychological function

This is an important area to enquire about, not only because dementia can cause a number of distressing psychological symptoms that should be picked up, but also because disturbances of psychological function may be the cause of the cognitive impairment (see Chapter 5). As a minimum, I cover possible symptoms of depression, anxiety (stress) and psychosis.

Depression symptoms
- Does the patient feel low in mood a lot of the time? Is it worse in the morning or the evening? Knowing this may help differentiate clinical depression from low mood associated with dementia; the former is classically associated with lower mood in the morning.
- Have they lacked 'get up and go'?
- Do they feel tired a lot of the time?
- Is their sleep disturbed? Do they have trouble getting off to sleep, or staying asleep? Do they wake up early in the morning and find they can't get back to sleep?
- What has their appetite been like? Have they lost or gained weight?
- Have they had trouble concentrating?
- Do they find little pleasure in things these days?
- Do they feel as though things are hopeless and won't get better?
- Do they feel worthless – as if they have no purpose?
- Do they sometimes feel like they'd be better off dead? Have they ever thought about ending their life? Would they

prefer to be dead? Do they feel like committing suicide? Do they have a plan? This is obviously a very important risk to recognise.

Anxiety symptoms
- Does the individual feel tense a lot of the time, like their muscles are all tight?
- Do they often feel as if they simply cannot cope?
- Do they find that they worry a lot about all sorts of things, including trivial matters?
- Have they noticed any other physical symptoms? This might include a lump in the throat, butterflies in the stomach, headaches, changes in breathing, a heightened awareness of their heartbeat, pins and needles in their hands, sweatiness or a tremor in the hands.
- Are there certain things that seem to trigger their anxiety? For example, interactions with people who they feel may be judging them, or feeling threatened in some way.
- Do they have times when their anxiety becomes so bad they think they might be going to die, have a heart attack or go mad? This may indicate panic attacks.
- Do they have trouble sleeping? Do they find it difficult to get off to sleep or to stay asleep?
- Do they feel tired a lot of the time?
- Are there things in their life that are causing them stress?
- Do they find they have to do things in a very particular way, or otherwise they get very stressed? Do they have any compulsions – things they feel they have to do over and over, and if they don't they feel anxious?
- Do they have thoughts that go around in their mind, thoughts they don't want but can't help having?

Psychotic symptoms
- Has the patient been worried about other people around them? Why is that?
- Do they feel threatened by anyone? Do they think others are trying to harm them in some way?

- Do they feel as if someone is set against them? Why would they?
- Have they been concerned about things going missing or being stolen? This is a very common belief in those with more moderate dementia; they may misplace objects, forget where they are and assume they have been taken.
- Have they heard people talking about them in a negative way? Can they see these people when they are doing so? What do they say?
- Has anything else unsettling or unexplainable happened to them lately?
- Have they seen anything they can't make sense of? Perhaps children running around, or animals?
- Do they believe they are special in some way, different from other people?
- Do they feel they are being controlled by someone or something? How would that work?
- Have they ever felt that people can hear their thoughts? Or that others can somehow extract thoughts from their brain? Or put thoughts directly into their head?
- Have they heard voices telling them to do things?

The discussion surrounding the possibility of a psychological cause of cognitive problems can involve a great deal more questioning. Sometimes, such problems can be quickly dismissed, though depression in particular is a condition that can mimic dementia – so-called *depressive pseudodementia* (see Chapter 5). Risk factors for a depressive component may include a previous history of depression, a strong family history of depression, or the presence of a *stressor* (a stressful life event) that seems to coincide with the cognitive problem developing. A patient's past psychiatric history – that is, any previous experience of mental health problems – is thus important to explore.

Physical function

Questions in this regard are often guided by what conditions the patient is known to have. Answers may indicate a potential cause for the cognitive problems, or a comorbid issue (in addition to the dementia) that needs to be dealt with.

- Has the individual felt unwell physically? In what way?
- Have they had trouble sleeping? Do they snore loudly or seem to have periods when they briefly stop breathing overnight? (This is a question for a bed-partner.) Do they wake with a headache? Do they feel exhausted throughout the day or fall asleep a lot during the day? This may indicate a condition called *obstructive sleep apnoea*.
- Have they felt sluggish, lacking in energy? Have they put on weight? Have they been unexpectedly constipated? Has their skin been dry? Has their face been puffy? These symptoms may indicate *thyroid disease*.
- Have they noticed that they are always thirsty or have a dry mouth? That they need to urinate more frequently than usual? Have they lost weight? Or felt weak and tired? Has their vision been blurred? Do they tend to heal slowly or seem prone to infections? All these could indicate *diabetes*.
- Have they had unexpected weight loss? Noticed blood in their stool or that their bowel habit is erratic? Do they cough up blood? Have there been any lumps in their skin that have not gone away or seem to be getting bigger? Has their voice become hoarse? Has there been blood in their urine? These symptoms, although quite non-specific, may raise the possibility of *cancer*.
- Do they drink more than the recommended amounts of alcohol? Is their diet poor? Do they feel weak? Are they constipated? Have they noticed numbness or tingling or problems when walking? A *vitamin B12 deficiency* can be the cause of these concerns.
- Have they had problems with incontinence? Had trouble focusing their eyes? Suffered with headaches? Have they been unsteady on their feet or had falls? Have they been drowsy? These symptoms can be associated with *hydrocephalus*.
- Have they had a sudden loss of vision or change in vision? Temporary or enduring changes in sensation or inexplicable increased pain in parts of their body? Urinary incontinence?

Have they felt very tired? Developed a tremor or had problems coordinating? Had poor balance? *Multiple sclerosis* needs to be considered as a diagnosis.

- Do they think they could be menopausal? Have they put on weight? Had unexplained mood swings? Hot flashes? Vaginal dryness? Suffered with insomnia? *Perimenopause*, although of course a normal phenomenon, may cause all these symptoms, as well as cognitive impairment.
- Are they known to have *cardiac disease*? Do they feel dizzy or light-headed often, especially when standing? Has their vision been blurred? Have they felt tired? Have they felt nauseated?
- Have they noticed increased fatigue, mood changes, bone pain, thinning hair? Have they had high blood pressure, frequent headaches, kidney stones, palpitations? *Abnormal calcium levels* and *hyperparathyroidism* need to be considered.
- Is there anything else they have been worried about in relation to their physical health?

It is important to note that the above symptoms are often non-specific (you will see that certain symptoms occur in a number of the health conditions) and are merely screening questions that may indicate the need for further consideration of the associated problems. Knowing a person's past medical history – for example, whether they have suffered heart disease, stroke, cancer – is therefore also of critical importance.

Medications

Have there been any changes in medication that are related in time to the onset of the cognitive problems? It surprises a lot of people how many commonly prescribed medications can cause problems with cognition, either by themselves or when used in combination. They may cause impairment either in someone who does not have dementia at all, or exacerbate underlying cognitive issues in someone who does have dementia.

A list of potentially problematic medications can be viewed on pages 65 and 66. This list is not exhaustive, and the use of the medications may not be relevant to the presenting concern of cognitive impairment – and of course they may be required for other conditions – but it is important to know what is being taken. Many medications may not cause problems by themselves, but if you are on a number of them at the same time the cumulative effect can be an issue. The two most common mechanisms behind the deleterious cognitive effects of medications are through their sedative and anticholinergic effects. As you may recall from Chapter 8, on Alzheimer's disease, the cholinergic system is critical for cognition, and anticholinergics interfere with this system.

It is also helpful to know whether there is a link in time between a medication being used and the cognitive impairment becoming evident as this may suggest *causality* – that the medication is the cause of the cognitive problems.

Substance use

Any centrally acting substance (one that affects the brain, either directly or indirectly) may have an effect on thinking, so it is important to understand what drugs a patient is using, whether legal (prescribed and over-the-counter) or illegal. A discussion around substance use should involve understanding the pattern of use of the following:

- Alcohol
- Marijuana
- Amphetamines such as dexamphetamine, methylphenidate, crystal methamphetamine (known as ice), speed and ecstasy
- Opiates such as heroin, morphine, buprenorphine, codeine and fentanyl

Most of these substances can cause a state of intoxication which causes an acute alteration in cognition, but their regular use over an extended period of time can also cause a chronic deficit in thinking which may not be reversible even with prolonged abstinence. (Regarding alcohol, see Chapter 9.)

Family history

A patient's family medical history may be relevant in highlighting an increased risk of dementia itself, or of an alternative medical condition that may mimic dementia (such as thyroid disease).

In the context of Alzheimer's disease, the relevance of a positive family history is greater with larger numbers of family members affected and with a younger age of onset. As we saw in Chapter 8, a family history of early-onset dementia, especially in more than one relative, is of considerable concern. Having one first-degree relative with late-onset dementia, however, does not greatly influence the absolute risk: advancing age plays much more of a role in this scenario.

Personal history

I try to gather as much of an individual's biographical history as possible. This involves looking at their life story. What was their childhood like? How did they get on with family and friends? How about their educational achievements and employment history? What have their intimate relationships been like? Have they experienced any major psychological traumas? How did they cope?

This may give hints as to the person's underlying personality style, vulnerabilities and coping mechanisms. What an individual experiences in life prior to the onset of dementia may greatly influence how the dementia affects them and how they may cope with the condition.

All the domains of history above need to be enquired about to a lesser or greater extent, depending on the responses given. Once I have obtained a full history, I am able to make some preliminary judgements about the nature and cause of the cognitive impairment.

Risk and legal issues

During the initial assessment, I also try to clarify certain other important issues:

- Has the patient threatened others or been verbally or physically aggressive to them? What was the context? This is a delicate issue, but can often be elucidated by discussing the natural frustrations that can come about with cognitive decline, and whether that has led to things getting out of control.
- Have there been any threats or concerns about deliberate self-harm?
- Is the person driving? Have they had any accidents? Is the carer more concerned than the patient? Poor insight into matters such as this is particularly concerning.
- Have they had any falls? What happened? Do they have a walking aid? Do they use it?
- Has a will been created? Has the patient formally written down their wishes about health interventions in the future? What about a substitute decision-maker? (See Chapter 21 for further information about these and other legal issues.)
- Has a My Aged Care assessment been performed (if in Australia)? What level of support has been funded?
- Does the patient want to stay where they are, or move into more supported accommodation?
- What does the patient want for their future? What does the carer want? This will help guide discussions around planning.

12

Physical Examination and Cognitive Testing

- A physical examination can reveal causes of cognitive impairment that are not dementia, or help clarify what type of dementia is present. It may also identify other problems that need to be addressed.
- Cognitive testing is an important part of assessing someone for dementia. It should be done in a quiet and relaxed space, and sensory deficits (such as hearing or vision issues) need to be taken into account.
- Performance anxiety may affect a person's ability to answer questions correctly, and this should be borne in mind.
- In tricky cases, referral to a neuropsychologist can be very helpful.

Once a patient's medical history has been gathered, and a list of *differential diagnoses* (the possible diagnoses) created, the next step is to examine the patient physically and perform some cognitive testing.

Physical examination

When it comes to physically examining a patient who has cognitive problems, certain areas are of particular relevance:

- *General level of alertness.* This may give a hint as to overuse of prescribed medications (or other drugs) or suggest acute ill health.
- *Any obvious evidence of infection.* Signs might include a high temperature, sweating, breathlessness or coughing (if the lungs are involved), cellulitis (inflammation of the skin characterised by redness, swelling and heat), and an offensive or strong smell in the urine (which may suggest a urinary tract infection). Infection can lead to a state of delirium, otherwise known as an acute confusional state. This may be the underlying cause of the cognitive impairment, or may be worsening the symptoms of a dementia that is also present.
- *Breathlessness or swelling of the lower limbs.* This may indicate heart failure, which can impair oxygenation of the brain.
- *Obvious signs of anaemia or dehydration.* These may include a dry tongue or lips, sunken eyes, reduced tissue turgor (fullness) and pale skin. Both of these conditions can lead to cognitive problems.
- *Body habitus* (shape). Although non-specific, how a person looks generally can give an indication of risk. Do they appear frail? Undernourished? Or are they overweight (in which case vascular disease, diabetes or sleep apnoea may be a concern)?
- *Blood pressure and pulse rate.* Elevated blood pressure (hypertension) and a fast or erratic/irregular pulse rate may indicate vascular disease, acute illness or thyroid disease (although so-called 'white coat hypertension' – the anxiety associated with attending the doctor – can also cause abnormal results). Low blood pressure in some can result in reduced blood flow to the brain and accentuate cognitive problems.
- *Gait* (or walking appearance). There are specific gait abnormalities that might give clues as to the underlying cause of cognitive impairment. These include the shuffling gait of Parkinson's disease and the broad-based gait of hydrocephalus or alcohol-related dementia (this is sometimes referred to as an *ataxic gait*). Walking may be slow due to Parkinson's disease or vascular subcortical disease. A *magnetic* gait – that is,

one with a wide base, and where the individual has trouble lifting their feet from the floor – is characteristic of frontal-lobe pathology. Walking may also elicit evidence of one-sided neurological damage that may be the result of a stroke; for example, swinging the leg outward and in a semicircle from the hip. Gait abnormalities are not a common feature of Alzheimer's disease in the early stages, and therefore may suggest a non-Alzheimer's cause. It is also important to consider the risk of falls when assessing gait.

- A *lump around the throat* (a goitre). This may suggest thyroid disease. Dry skin and puffiness in the face may also occur with low thyroid function.

Certain other neurological signs may be present:

- Other *features of Parkinson's disease* may be evident, such as a tremor in the hands, increased tone in the limb muscles and 'cogwheeling' in the arms (the arms move in 'steps' rather than smoothly when they are passively moved, as if the different sections have cogs connecting them). As noted previously, parkinsonism can occur for a number of reasons – not only Parkinson's disease, but also other subcortical diseases. It may also be related to medications the patient is on.
- *Myoclonus* – involuntary jerking of the limbs – may be seen in Huntington's disease and dementia with Lewy bodies, though also in Alzheimer's disease. It may also be reflective of an underlying epilepsy.
- *Abnormal eye movements* may accompany alcohol-related damage and a Parkinson's-like condition known as *progressive supranuclear palsy*, though these are often non-specific.
- *Asymmetry of facial features* (when one side appears different to the other) may indicate a previous stroke.
- *Asymmetry of power and sensation*, especially in the upper or lower limb, may also suggest a stroke.
- *Slurred speech* (dysarthria) can also occur due to a stroke. *Soft speech* (hypophonia) is suggestive of Parkinson's disease.

If certain other conditions are suspected – such as heart disease or diabetes – further physical examinations may need to be done. The examination may also pick up other problems not associated with the dementia, but which need to be taken into account. Problems with mobilising – leading to an increased risk of falls – are a good example: this may influence the choice of medication used going forward.

Cognitive testing

Once it has been established that cognitive impairment is present, the next step is to get an idea of the specific deficits, and we do this by testing the various cognitive domains. This may help illuminate the cause of the cognitive problems, as well as specific problems that may need to be addressed.

Before commencing any cognitive test, it is important that the patient feels as comfortable as possible. I often preface the assessment by acknowledging that they have been put 'on the spot' – that it is natural for them to feel anxious, and that this may impact their performance in the test. It is also important to emphasise that the cognitive tests are only part of the puzzle; the results do not, in and of themselves, confirm any diagnosis.

I try to ensure that the room in which the test is conducted is quiet, brightly lit and free of distractions, and that the individual can hear and see properly. If they cannot, that needs to be taken into consideration; certain tests may not then be appropriate to perform.

It is my preference that the carer/person accompanying the patient stays in the room while we conduct the test – as long as they do not help or give clues/answers to the questions being asked! Their witnessing of the testing can be quite helpful when we discuss the details later. In order to minimise anxiety, however, I usually ask the patient whether they would prefer to do it by themselves or with their carer present.

Standardised cognitive tests
The Mini-Mental State Examination (MMSE), created by Marshal Folstein in the 1970s, is one of the most recognised and commonly

used cognitive tests, and is often performed by a patient's GP before the patient is referred to me. It has the advantage of only taking a few minutes to conduct, and its familiarity means that most medical practitioners can easily recognise the level of impairment from the score. It has certain disadvantages, such as not testing executive function well, and only really picking up more advanced short-term memory difficulties. Those with high premorbid IQ can also blitz the MMSE despite having early dementia, and it can therefore be falsely reassuring. A score below 24 out of 30 is generally considered to represent significant cognitive impairment.

Another test of similar brevity is the Montreal Cognitive Assessment (MoCA). This was originally designed to help differentiate between mild cognitive impairment and dementia, acknowledging the poor sensitivity of the MMSE in doing this. The test of short-term memory is slightly harder, and there is a little executive function testing incorporated. It is also scored out of 30, with 22 being the average score for someone with mild cognitive impairment. A score of 18 or below is often seen as suggestive of dementia.

One of the challenges with most cognitive tests is that they skew towards those who have English as their first language; those who do not speak the language well may achieve falsely low scores. In response to this problem, another brief test, the Rowland Universal Dementia Assessment Scale, or RUDAS, has been developed. It has been translated into a number of other language versions. Like the MoCA and MMSE, it is brief and scored out of 30. A score of 22 or less is considered abnormal.

Although I have not personally used it, a well-validated cognitive screening test has been developed for assessing older Indigenous Australians. This is the Kimberley Indigenous Cognitive Assessment, or KICA.

My preference when assessing cognition in my clinic is to use one of the versions of Addenbrooke's Cognitive Examination (ACE), a longer test that takes about 20 minutes to complete but which can give a clearer sense of frontal (executive) problems, as well as testing short-term memory more rigorously. It covers most cognitive domains and has evidence to suggest it can differentiate between frontotemporal dementia and Alzheimer's dementia (by delineating the relative impairment on language and executive tests vs memory tests). It is scored out of 100, with a nominal cut-off of 83/100.

In some instances, I also use the Hopkins Verbal Learning Test (HVLT). This specifically tests the ability to remember information provided verbally (verbal memory). A list of 12 words is read out and the patient is asked to recall as many of them as they can immediately afterwards. The list is then read out twice more, and the patient is asked to recall what they remember after each time. The scores are then compared to averages for the population ('norms') to see if there is a significant difference. It is hoped that with each trial, more items are recalled, confirming the ability for *new learning*. After three trials, another list of words is read aloud, some of which are in the original list and some not. The patient is then asked to state whether they were in the list. If the patient cannot spontaneously recall the words (with the three trials) but correctly identifies them when they are called out, this suggests a problem of retrieval rather than acquisition, potentially helping determine the type of dementia present. The HVLT is considerably more sensitive in picking up early short-term memory deficits than the ACE or MMSE.

Numerous other tests of memory and cognition are available. The Neuropsychiatry Unit Cognitive Assessment Tool (known as NUCOG), developed by the Neuropsychiatry Unit of Royal Melbourne Hospital, deserves an honourable mention. There is no one perfect test, however. They all have advantages and disadvantages. Although I have my own favoured assessments, many others will be equally valuable. The point is to try to get a good sense of what areas of cognition – orientation, memory (short-term and long-term), language, praxis, calculation, visuospatial and executive ability – are affected. This knowledge may suggest a particular diagnosis, and also has implications for how a person's day-to-day function may be affected.

Other specific tests of cognitive function

I often pursue several specific lines of enquiry as I attempt to diagnose the cause of an apparent cognitive loss:

- Problems with *orientation* are easily demonstrated by asking the individual where they are exactly (in which clinic, on what floor, in which city, state and country) and what day, date, month, year and season it is. Orientation is usually covered in the formal tests detailed above, however.
- Problems with *working memory* can be determined by asking the patient to recall an increasing sequence of numbers, both forward and backward.
- Problems with *short-term memory* may be informally demonstrated by asking what the patient may have done that morning or afternoon, or what they had to eat and so on. Having an informant present to corroborate the information is vital.
- Problems with *language* can be elicited by asking an individual to name familiar objects, to read words aloud or to repeat unusual phrases. Again, these are incorporated into some of the tests above.
- Problems with *praxis* can be elicited by asking individuals to copy drawings or to mime the use of everyday objects – for example, brushing their teeth or brushing their hair. Those with mild problems often can demonstrate the movement but use their own finger as the brush, rather than miming that they are holding the brush.

Further tests of executive function

To get a better sense of executive function, I often ask a patient to complete a number of other tasks. These include the *Luria two-step* and *three-step tests*, both of which involve copying a sequence of hand movements that I perform. This in part demonstrates whether an individual can change *cognitive set* (that is, whether they can shift from one type of thinking – here manifest as a certain hand position – to another). Individuals with executive problems may simply repeat the same movement rather than change to the others in the sequence.

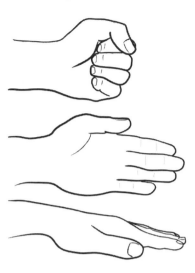

The Luria three-step test. Individuals are asked to repeat the sequence of hand movements above.

A *tapping test* assesses the ability to inhibit impulses, another executive function. This involves asking the patient to tap twice when I tap once, and to tap once when I tap twice. Impaired individuals may simply copy the number of taps I perform.

Completing a sequence of alternating shapes may also reveal problems; again, this demonstrates an inability to shift cognitively from one shape to the next.

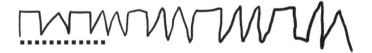

Alternating square and triangle task. Note the repetition of the triangle shape.

Interestingly, asking individuals about the meaning of proverbs (such as 'a rolling stone gathers no moss') can also highlight frontal-lobe problems. If these are present, responses tend to be concrete: a response to the rolling stone proverb may be 'It means that a stone doesn't get any moss on it if it is always rolling,' rather than 'Someone who is always moving doesn't pick up responsibilities and cares.' This is due to problems with abstract thinking. The cultural background of the patient needs to be taken into account when using this test, however, as proverbs are inherently specific to the culture in which they arise.

Neuropsychological assessment

With a selection of results from the above tests, as well as the patient's medical history, it is usually possible to get a preliminary idea about what may be going on – both the nature and the severity of the problem. There are times, however, when the situation remains unclear despite all the consultation-room testing. In this case, referral to a neuropsychologist can be very helpful. These are professionals who have general training in psychology, but also specific training in assessing cognition.

Assessments made by neuropsychologists are considerably more involved and time-consuming – sometimes they're done over a number of hours, and over different sessions – but they really are the gold standard of cognitive testing. They can be particularly helpful in early cases of dementia and when testing those with high premorbid IQ, as they may sail through the consultation-room testing displaying no obvious problems. Unfortunately, in Australia, a visit to a neuropsychologist is not funded by Medicare, so it can be quite expensive. Neuropsychologists are often part of the team in a publicly funded memory clinic, however, in which case there may be no cost.

13

Investigations

- Investigations are an important part of the work-up of cognitive problems.
- There are a number of standard blood and urine tests that should be conducted as part of the investigations.
- A structural brain scan – ideally an MRI scan – should be performed if possible. In some cases, functional brain scans, which show real-time activity in the brain, can also aid the process of diagnosis.
- A number of investigations that are currently used primarily in research hold promise for better detection of early dementia in the future.

Once the history, physical examination and cognitive testing have been completed, it is time to consider what investigations need to be performed. These tests and scans are an important part of the process, as they may help identify reversible causes of cognitive impairment. They may also support a provisional diagnosis of a form of dementia that has already been made. Finally, they may identify other conditions that could complicate the treatment of symptoms of dementia.

Investigations can be divided into blood and urine tests, neuroimaging (brain scans), and other selected tests.

Blood and urine tests

Many of these will have already been completed by the referring GP, though I like to ensure that the following blood tests have been done:

- *Full blood count.* We are looking in particular for signs of anaemia or infection.
- *Sodium levels.* Low sodium, which may be due to a number of medical and medication-related problems, is a common cause of confusion.
- *Renal (kidney) function.* If impaired, this can lead to *uraemia* due to impaired clearance of urea, which may cause cognitive problems. As many medications are excreted by the kidneys, reduced function can also impact their effectiveness and safety.
- *Hepatic (liver) function.* Hepatic impairment can also affect cognition. Testing of liver enzymes may show a history of alcohol misuse, which can also contribute to cognitive problems.
- *Calcium and parathyroid hormone.* Abnormalities of calcium and the parathyroid gland may cause impairment of thinking.
- *Thyroid function.* Disordered thyroid function can affect cognition, both directly and through its effect on mood. Low thyroid function, in particular, is associated with depression.
- *Vitamin B12 and folate.* These minerals are critical for brain health, and a deficiency may be the cause of the cognitive problems. (See Chapter 3 for more information.)
- *Vitamin D.* Research suggests an association between low vitamin D levels and dementia. (See Chapter 4 for more information.)
- *Homocysteine.* Elevated levels have been associated with an increased risk of vascular disease and Alzheimer's pathology in particular. (See Chapter 8 for more information.)
- *Fasting blood sugar and cholesterol.* These are important to identify as risk factors for vascular disease, such as pre-diabetes and diabetes. Marked fluctuations in blood sugar in and of themselves can also cause acute changes in cognition.

- *Inflammatory markers.* These include c-reactive protein and erythrocyte sedimentation rate and indicate there may be inflammation in the body. Raised inflammatory markers are non-specific but can indicate a covert problem that could be contributing to cognitive problems.
- *HIV and syphilis.* Although there is some controversy about routinely testing for these two infectious diseases (as they are very uncommon), they are important not to miss as both can cause dementia-type illnesses.

I also like to make sure a *urine microscopy and culture* has been completed. Infections of the urinary tract are a common contributor to cognitive problems, especially in the elderly. They may be the cause of confusion by themselves, but more commonly are responsible for exacerbating the cognitive impairment seen in those with dementia.

Neuroimaging

Unless there is certainty about a particular reversible cause of cognitive impairment, neuroimaging is an essential investigation. This involves performing scans to assess the structure and/or functioning of the brain.

There are two types of *structural brain scan* that are commonly performed: the *computed tomography* (CT) scan, and the *magnetic resonance imaging* (MRI) scan.

CT scan
CT scans use radiation at a low dose to visualise the structure of the brain. They have the advantage of being cheap and relatively quick to perform. The individual lies on a narrow moving bed that enters a scanner, which has the form of a large ring. It tends to be a quiet process, and most people find that the space does not seem too small. The scan may only take five minutes to perform.

CT scans can demonstrate more obvious abnormal features of the brain, including tumours, extensive vascular disease or atrophy (shrinkage). Their resolution (the ability to pick out detail) is considerably less than that of an MRI, however, and so important details may not be clear. For this reason, I always like to obtain an MRI if it is feasible.

MRI scan

These scans are obtained with a machine that uses powerful magnets to move protons (positively charged subatomic particles) in such a way as to create a well-defined image of whatever they are scanning.

Similarly to a CT scan, having an MRI brain scan also involves being placed on a moving bed that enters a ring-shaped scanner, though the space tends to be considerably smaller and those with claustrophobia can become a little anxious (premedication with light sedatives is sometimes helpful). It is also a noisy process, though the patient is usually given earplugs. An MRI can also take considerably longer than a CT scan to complete (perhaps up to 30 minutes). If a patient has metal in their body, or a pacemaker, it is important to consider whether this will be affected by the scanner. Unfortunately, in Australia MRI scans are less accessible than CT scans.

Scan results

Whether the patient has had a CT scan or an MRI scan or both, there are four aspects that are commonly relevant to the investigation of cognitive impairment:

- *Head injury*. These may result in haemorrhages (abnormal collections of blood on or in the brain), which are usually evident on both types of scan.
- *Atrophy (shrinkage)*. This may be *global* (the whole brain) or *localised* (where shrinkage is much more obvious in certain areas).
- *Vascular disease*. There may be evidence of small or large strokes.
- *Brain tumour*. These are uncommon, though nonetheless important to rule out.

Both CT and MRI scans visualise the brain in different *planes* (angles): from front to back, from left to right, and from top to bottom. When there is a suspicion of Alzheimer's disease, I find that *coronal slices* – those from the front to the back of the brain – are especially helpful, as they most clearly demonstrate the volume of the hippocampi and surrounding tissues. Shrinkage of these areas in someone who fits the clinical profile of having Alzheimer's disease is a strong indication that this is the underlying problem. Those with different types of dementia – for instance, frontotemporal dementia – may have disproportionate shrinkage in other areas (see Chapter 9).

Interpretation of structural brain scans can be a somewhat subjective process. In most cases, a radiologist (a medical doctor who specialises in interpreting these scans) will provide an opinion as to the extent of atrophy and vascular disease, and comment on whether it is an amount that would normally be seen for a person of that age. With increasing age (perhaps starting about age 60), there is usually a noticeable degree of shrinkage and vascular disease, and it can sometimes be hard to determine whether the presence of either of these changes is normal for age or more than expected (and so perhaps related to a disease process like Alzheimer's). Despite this limitation, however, neuroimaging is an important part of the process of diagnosing someone with a possible dementia.

Other brain scans

In some cases, I also rely on *functional neuroimaging*. These scans show the *activity* of different parts of the brain while the patient is in the scanner. Broadly speaking, there are three types of functional imaging:

- *Single-photon emission computed tomography* (SPECT) scans. These show regional blood flow in the brain, an indicator of potential damage.
- *Positron emission tomography* (PET) scans. These reveal glucose (sugar) metabolism in the brain in real time. Areas of reduced metabolism suggest damage to that part of the brain.
- *Functional MRI* (fMRI) scans. Like SPECT scans, these measure regional blood flow.

It can be particularly helpful to correlate the findings of a structural and a functional scan. For example, someone who has subtle shrinkage of their frontal and temporal lobes may have corresponding reduced activity on their functional scan. This may then support a diagnosis of frontotemporal dementia.

There are two issues with functional neuroimaging, however. One is accessibility: although SPECT scans are reasonably available, PET scans and fMRI scans can be quite hard to obtain outside major urban centres. The other issue is the lack of detail and specificity of the findings: the ability of these scans (and in particular SPECT scans) to pick up subtle changes in activity that may be clinically relevant is limited. Nonetheless, functional neuroimaging can sometimes be a helpful addition to the diagnostic process.

Other investigations

In some cases, further investigations may be appropriate. If there is evidence of vascular disease, an ultrasound scan of the carotid arteries in the neck (a *carotid doppler*) may be performed, looking for narrowing of the vessels due to a build-up of plaque. If there are concerns about epilepsy, chronic delirium or encephalitis, an *electroencephalogram* (or EEG) may be worthwhile. This involves placing multiple sensors, attached to a helmet, over the head, and recording the electrical activity of the brain.

If an atypical dementia (that is, one that does not fit the profile of the commoner types) is suspected in a younger individual, and especially if it is associated with prominent neurological features, a *lumbar puncture* may be worth undertaking (if this is the case, I involve a neurologist). In this procedure, a thin needle is used to draw cerebrospinal fluid from the lower spine. This fluid is then sent to a lab for analysis.

Further investigations used primarily in research

It is worth mentioning here a few other investigative procedures that may be helpful in determining whether someone has (or is at risk of developing) dementia. The first involves a specialised type of PET scan in which a patient is injected with a chemical (a ligand) that binds to amyloid or tau, revealing its presence in the brain. This can be helpful in detecting the presence of *pre-clinical* Alzheimer's disease – that is, where there are no signs or symptoms of the disease but there is evidence of underlying brain tissue pathology. In Australia at least, such scans are generally used only in research facilities.

There are a number of other biological markers (or biomarkers) of the Alzheimer's disease process. Their presence can be detected most reliably in the cerebrospinal fluid (obtained through a lumbar puncture, as mentioned earlier). Beta-amyloid and tau can both be detected, as can other markers of inflammation or infection. In some parts of the world, lumbar punctures are already being used to aid diagnosis, though in Australia this is currently not routine. As noted in Chapter 8, a blood test for tau shows considerable promise for very early detection of Alzheimer's disease.

Biomarkers are a growing field, and may be of great value clinically in the future. In Australia, the CSIRO is currently engaged in a large, long-term study, part of whose aim is to identify useful biomarkers. This is the Australian Imaging, Biomarker and Lifestyle flagship study of ageing.

In the next section of the book, we will explore significant physical, psychological and behavioural aspects of life for those who have been diagnosed with dementia.

SECTION II

After a Diagnosis

14

Coping with the News

- Being told you have dementia can evoke a spectrum of emotions, which is normal and expected. These may fluctuate considerably.

- Sometimes, receiving a diagnosis of a form of dementia can be a relief, as it provides an explanation for what has been happening. It also allows plans to be made.

- Grief is a common emotional response, and may be in anticipation of future losses.

- Seeking the support of others can be of great help emotionally.

- For some, the news can cause clinical depression or anxiety. It is important to recognise the signs and seek help from a professional if required.

Receiving a diagnosis of Alzheimer's disease, vascular dementia or another type of dementia can be a very harrowing experience – both for the individual with the condition and for their carers or loved ones. As a clinician, I have to judge how much detail to give when breaking the news, acknowledging that some individuals want to know everything, while others would rather not hear anything. I am also conscious that the person receiving the news can 'switch off' – because of the shock of the diagnosis or because too much information is given, or both.

Through experience, however, I also know that many individuals and their carers have anticipated that dementia is likely before I even confirm it – after all, they have been living with the problem for some time, and dementia as a concept is widely known. As a result, sometimes a patient, carer or loved one feels a sense of relief when they are given the diagnosis. At last they have an explanation for the difficulties they have been experiencing, even if the reason is not what they hoped. Knowing what the issue is at least allows them to make plans to deal with it.

Emotional responses to a dementia diagnosis

Despite the remarkable capacity of many to deal with a diagnosis, there are numerous emotional responses that signify distress. These include shock and disbelief, numbness, denial, anger, hopelessness, despair and pervasive sadness. Individuals may oscillate from one emotional state to another, feeling as if they're on an emotional roller-coaster. All these responses are normal and understandable. One heartening truth is that, for most, these negative emotions do improve with time as they accept the diagnosis and focus instead on what they can do to improve their situation.

For the carer or loved one, a phenomenon known as *anticipatory grief* may develop: this is when they grieve for anticipated losses in the future. A process known as *ambiguous grief* may also occur, where the grief seems misplaced because the individual is still alive and present. Grieving in this instance develops because of the absence and loss of the normal psychological and emotional connection one had with the person experiencing dementia. It is important to recognise that these emotions, as with many of the others that people feel, are a normal part of dealing with a dementia diagnosis.

Although the above responses may be normal, their impact can be lessened if those trying to cope reach out for the support of others. Having someone to talk to, even if just to 'vent', can be invaluable. Sometimes the simplest of warm interactions can change the way we feel about the situation and make us feel less alone.

A number of other strategies may be of help if you are seeking to manage your emotional response. These include: acknowledging and accepting your feelings rather than holding them inside;

managing stress and tension by allowing yourself to cry, or even by punching pillows (away from others); and ensuring there are other things in your life that do not revolve around the illness and its implications. Scheduling pleasurable activities can be a helpful strategy. If you are a carer, it is very important to make time for yourself. Peer support – getting to know others who are going through similar experiences – can be invaluable and make you feel less alone. It is still possible to have fun and enjoy life with someone experiencing the symptoms of dementia: despite the expected cognitive decline, much of what you have loved about the person may remain for many years.

It is important to recognise, however, when your response to being informed of dementia morphs into something more. The risk of developing a clinical depression, or an anxiety disorder, is higher in the aftermath of a dementia diagnosis, both for the person experiencing the condition and for their carers or loved ones. If there is any doubt about this, you should seek the help of your GP or a counsellor. If you experience persistent changes in your sleep pattern or appetite, or if you feel that everything is bleak and hopeless, or especially if you feel as if life is not worth living, then it is critical that you talk to someone. The stress of being a carer, too, can complicate the emotional response. Chapter 23 provides more detail on managing carer stress.

What next?

What happens after you are given a diagnosis of dementia? This depends to a large extent on what has occurred beforehand, but there are a number of issues that may need to be looked at. These include the issue of driving, as well as legal ramifications and advanced care planning; we'll look at these in detail in Chapter 21. Receiving a diagnosis should generate a discussion about whether the current supports are adequate, and about what can be accessed now or in the future (see Chapter 23).

Education about the condition can be invaluable. This is of course one of the main purposes of this book, and the following chapters describe some of the main changes and challenges to expect with dementia. There are also some fantastic websites dedicated to dementia education and support; often these are run by organisations that can provide carer education sessions and support. Refer to the Appendix for more information.

Treatment of dementia encompasses a number of different domains. These may include treatment of the cognitive loss itself, as well as treatment of any associated risk factors, such as vascular disease. It may also involve treatment of non-cognitive problems that may arise, be they psychological, physical or behavioural. Management of dementia also involves optimising communication and finding purpose and meaning despite the losses. Understanding and addressing the impact of caring for someone with a chronic, progressive condition is also crucial: carers are often the 'hidden victims' of the disease, and their needs regularly go unmet.

Let's look first at what we can do about the cognitive effects of dementia.

15

Management of Cognitive Loss

- There are a number of lifestyle interventions that may help slow the rate of cognitive decline. They are better put in place earlier rather than later.

- External memory aids and mental strategies can be very helpful for some in the earlier stages of dementia.

- There are medications for cognitive loss in dementia. These treatments are not curative but can alleviate symptoms, slow the rate of cognitive decline and improve day-to-day function, especially in the early stages. They may be especially helpful when Alzheimer's disease is the cause of the dementia.

- Cholinesterase inhibitors generally work by increasing the amount of acetylcholine – a neurotransmitter – between nerve cells.

- Memantine works on another neurotransmitter, glutamate, and may be more beneficial in later stages of dementia.

It is everyone's hope that, over the next decade, we will find a cure for dementia. Until that time, however, our aim is to preserve, as best we can, what cognitive capacity an individual has.

As we have seen, one of the defining features of dementia is its progressive course. With or without medication, the expected trajectory of the underlying disease is of increasing cognitive and functional decline. The medications we have at our disposal cannot reverse the damage done by the disease; their intention is to allow us to make the most of what is left. This, for some, can mean a noticeable improvement in thinking and function, while for others it may mean that the rate of further decline is slowed.

General interventions

It is worth noting, before we embark on a discussion about medications, that there are some general recommendations that may help to preserve cognition in someone with dementia, especially if it is caught early. As we saw in Chapter 3, these include:

- Exercising regularly and staying physically fit
- Eating well
- Ensuring vascular health is optimised
- Socialising with others (socialising is a cognitive task and exercises the brain, and there is validity to the idea of 'use it or lose it')
- Ensuring that the brain is taxed regularly (exercising the brain by completing puzzles and other cognitive activities may be of some benefit, as long as it is not too stressful or frustrating)
- Optimising hearing.

Although these interventions may be most powerful as a preventative against dementia – and therefore are best started before the condition develops – they are unlikely to do any harm once the condition has occurred, and for some may be beneficial.

Environmental changes

There are a number of environmental and behavioural interventions that may lessen the impact of memory loss in particular.

- Using external memory aids can be of great benefit. These may come in the form of shopping lists or message boards in the home.
- It can also be helpful to use a diary and/or a calendar, and to ensure that everything important is written down. Carers can

encourage this and remind the individual with the condition to refer to this regularly. The diary or calendar should be positioned in an easily visible place.

- An alarm – either on a clock or a mobile phone (as long as it can be easily located) – can be useful for reminding an individual to take their medications or to keep scheduled appointments.
- Sticky notes in visible places such as the fridge can also be helpful reminders.
- There are electronic tags with in-built GPS that can be attached to items that are frequently misplaced, such as wallets and keys. These tags play a sound when a locator device is pressed.

Mental strategies

Most individuals who receive a dementia diagnosis still retain some capacity for new learning in the early stages of the disease. We do not go from having a good memory one day to not being able to recall anything the next. Especially in the early stages of the disease, therefore, certain mental strategies for remembering can be of benefit:

- Breaking up lists or numbers into clumps of three or four items/numbers makes recall easier.
- Actively testing yourself on what has been learnt helps cement the information in the mind, and can make it easier to recall later on.
- The use of mnemonics and stories can be beneficial. Rhymes, songs, acronyms or amusing mental images can be very helpful as memory aids.
- Minimising distractions while attempting to learn new information makes the process easier.

All these measures are more appropriate for those who have only mild symptoms of dementia. I often advise patients to try several different strategies and see which one works best for them. It is also important that mental strategies and other interventions do not induce stress, as this is likely to be counterproductive.

As dementia progresses, memory aids and mental strategies may be of less benefit. As this occurs, one of the most helpful interventions is to try to keep a routine that is familiar and predictable. Orienting individuals with calendars and clocks may still be of some benefit, and reading a daily paper or watching the news may also help. This can also be a good way of promoting conversations that orient us in 'real' life.

Medications

Alzheimer's disease

Currently, there are four licensed medications to treat the cognitive symptoms of Alzheimer's disease. Three influence the *cholinergic system* and are known as *cholinesterase inhibitors*. The other works through modulating the *glutamatergic system*. Both systems are thought to be damaged in Alzheimer's disease.

Cholinesterase inhibitors

These include *donepezil, rivastigmine* and *galantamine*. Note that these are the generic names; these medications are off-patent and therefore have numerous brand names. As we saw in Chapter 9, our theories regarding Alzheimer's disease suggest there is a deficit in acetylcholine, a chemical responsible for facilitating transmission between different neurons in the brain. Cholinesterase inhibitors work by inhibiting the enzyme (cholinesterase) that breaks down this chemical between the nerve cells. The net effect is that the amount of acetylcholine between the nerve cells is increased and there is increased connectivity between the nerve cells. The connectivity is what underpins our cognitive abilities.

It should be noted that these medications do not 'treat' the underlying disease per se – the amount of amyloid and tau remains unchanged – but they do give symptomatic relief for some by raising the level of the abnormally depleted neurotransmitter. In this, they are rather like oil in a machine that helps it run more efficiently.

Cholinesterase inhibitors demonstrate a modest but noticeable effect in some patients with certain types of dementia due to Alzheimer's disease. These medications only work as long as they are taken, and within a few weeks of ceasing them the symptoms will return to how they were before treatment.

Studies show that the greatest cognitive benefit of cholinesterase inhibitors occurs in those in the milder stages of Alzheimer's disease, and this underpins the importance of recognising and treating the illness early on. They can be an important part of the process undertaken to keep individuals with dementia at home for as long as possible. This, for many, is one of the most important objectives to achieve.

Cholinesterase inhibitors can also favourably influence the neuropsychiatric features of dementia, both early on and sometimes in more severe stages of the disease. These difficulties, also known as the *behavioural and psychological symptoms of dementia*, can be the most troublesome aspects of the disease; we'll discuss these in the following chapters.

Decisions about using these medications is influenced not only by the severity and nature of the dementia, but also by the potential for side effects. There are three specific conditions that can be exacerbated by the use of cholinesterase inhibitors:

- *Chronic restrictive airways disease*, such as chronic obstructive pulmonary disease (COPD), emphysema and asthma
- *Gastric ulcers* (especially if active)
- *Cardiac problems* that may cause a slow heart rate, such as heart block or sick sinus syndrome.

Due to the modest benefits of cholinesterase inhibitors, they are best not used in individuals in whom any of these three conditions are problematic. For the first two illnesses, it is usually evident whether there is a problem from the history or examination, but cardiac vulnerabilities can be *silent* (that is, one can have a problem and not know about it). For this reason, performing an electrocardiogram (ECG) is an important part of the 'work-up' for an individual who may be starting a cholinesterase inhibitor. This is a simple and painless test that involves having a few sticky dots applied to the chest. These are attached to leads that register the electrical activity of the heart, revealing any evidence of conduction disturbance and/or slow heart rate. If there is any uncertainty from the ECG about whether cholinesterase will be suitable from a cardiac perspective, a referral to a specialist in the area (a cardiologist) may be warranted.

On the whole, cholinesterase inhibitors are relatively well tolerated. Some individuals report gastrointestinal symptoms (nausea, vomiting and diarrhoea), headaches, sleep difficulties, fatigue and/or a degree of agitation. Weight loss can also occur, as can muscle pain (myalgia). These side effects are usually mild and often disappear after a few days or a week or so. Sometimes there is a paradoxical worsening of cognition, with increased confusion. If the side effects are severe or persist, the medication is usually stopped. If this does occur, it may be worth a trial of one of the other cholinesterase inhibitors; although the drugs are in the same class, some individuals seem to tolerate one but not another. If an individual does not tolerate two agents in this class, however, I tend to not try the third.

It can take some time for patients to respond to cholinesterase inhibitors, and it is usual to reassess cognition only after a number of months of being on a therapeutic dose of the medication. In Australia, an initial six-month supply is subsidised by the government. If there is evidence during this time that the medication has been helpful, the government will subsidise ongoing use.

The response to cholinesterase inhibitors is often more qualitative than quantitative. That is to say, improvements may be hard to measure exactly, though the individual and/or their carer feel that they generally function better from day to day. Although formal cognitive testing may not demonstrate the improvement, these qualitative reports are important to consider. Changes may be in the form of improved retention and memory, or more generally with regard to the activities of daily living. There may also be some benefit in terms of mood, irritability and anxiety.

Rivastigmine is the only cholinesterase inhibitor that comes in the form of a patch, and this is the one that I tend to favour initially. My experience suggests that transdermal patches are better tolerated (that is, they produce fewer side effects), perhaps related to the slow release of the medication. They also have the advantage in cases where swallowing tablets is difficult. The patch needs to be changed daily. Some individuals may develop a local reaction to the patch, such as a rash, in which case one of the oral forms can be tried.

There is no compelling evidence to suggest significant differences in effectiveness between the three cholinesterase inhibitors when it comes to treating Alzheimer's disease. In my practice, therefore, the choice of agent depends primarily on tolerability.

As with most medications, cholinesterase inhibitors should be started at a low dose to ensure they are tolerated, and 'up-titrated' (the dose increased) according to evidence of effectiveness and tolerability.

Medication	Starting dose	Dose increase schedule	Maximum dose
Donepezil (tablet)	5 mg daily	May increase to 10 mg once daily after one month	10 mg daily
Rivastigmine (capsule/oral solution)	1.5 mg twice daily	May increase by 1.5 mg (twice daily) every two weeks	6 mg twice daily
Rivastigmine (skin patch)	4.6 mg/ 24 hours	May increase to 13.3 mg/24 hours with time	13.3 mg/ 24 hours
Galantamine extended release (capsule)	8 mg daily	May increase to 16 mg daily after four weeks, then 24 mg daily after another four weeks.	24 mg daily

Dosage schedule for cholinesterase inhibitors.

Opinions about when to stop cholinesterase inhibitors vary. Given that their effectiveness in treating cognitive impairment seems restricted to the mild stages of the disease, and that a large part of their usefulness is in maintaining function so that the individual can stay in their home for as long as possible, there is an argument that they should be stopped once the individual enters supported care (such as an aged-care facility). The same argument could be made when the disease has advanced to the moderate or severe stages. We do know that they can also be helpful in treating the behavioural and psychological symptoms of dementia during these later stages, however, and if I am concerned about these I may keep the medications going beyond the point at which the cognitive advantages usually disappear.

The response to cholinesterase inhibitors can be divided into three categories. The most optimistic outcome is that memory function improves (beyond what it was like when not on the medications) *and* the progression of symptoms slows. Approximately one third of patients may respond in this way. Another third show no obvious immediate improvement in cognition, but the progression of symptoms slows. The last third of patients, unfortunately, derive no obvious benefit.

Memantine

This medication works primarily by blocking NMDA receptors, a subtype of glutamate receptor that exists on neurons. Glutamate, like acetylcholine, is a neurotransmitter, but it facilitates transmission of messages in the glutamatergic system as opposed to the cholinergic system. In high doses, however, glutamate appears to be toxic to the brain. Memantine is thought to protect nerve cells from being overstimulated by glutamate. It does so by occupying the receptors that the glutamate would otherwise attach to, reducing the amount of glutamate-related damage.

Like the cholinesterase inhibitors, memantine has not been shown to stop or reverse the damage wrought by whatever condition is causing the dementia, but it does seem to help improve the cognitive (and non-cognitive) symptoms of Alzheimer's disease. Memantine's role in treating dementia is generally regarded as being relevant in the later stages of the disease; in Australia, it is licensed for use in cases of moderate to severe dementia. I do sometimes prescribe it in the milder phases, however, either when cholinesterase inhibitors cannot be used or as an adjunct to those. The Australian government only subsidises either memantine or cholinesterase inhibitors, not both, so memantine is often written as a private script; being off-patent, it is not terribly expensive. As they work in different ways, there are no major interactional issues.

Memantine has the advantage of being relatively well tolerated, though more common side effects include fatigue, headaches, body aches, dizziness and constipation. In some it may induce hallucinations and can increase confusion. Similarly to cholinesterase inhibitors, these problems tend to be mild and may disappear as the body gets used to the drug. In my experience, memantine can be helpful in treating problematic or distressing psychiatric symptoms in individuals with dementia. As these often arise in the later stages of the disease, it can be a useful option if medications are required.

Memantine is initially prescribed at a dose of 5 milligrams per day, and the dose is increased by 5-milligram increments each week until the therapeutic dose of 20 milligrams per day is reached. Like the cholinesterase inhibitors, it can take many weeks (up to 12) for a therapeutic effect to develop.

Vascular dementia

Certain studies have demonstrated that cholinesterase inhibitors may improve cognition in vascular dementia, an idea that makes sense considering we know that vascular disease may damage the cholinergic system. However, the majority of specialists tend to agree that the role of cholinesterase inhibitors is less certain in this disease compared to Alzheimer's disease. There is, in my experience, often an overlap between Alzheimer's disease and vascular dementia (known as *mixed dementia*), however, and in these cases a trial of a cholinesterase inhibitor seems very reasonable.

The evidence for using memantine to treat vascular dementia is not especially compelling, though the studies that have been done suggest there may be small benefits for cognitive function (as well as for behaviour and mood symptoms).

The treatment of the cognitive problems in vascular dementia is primarily focused on trying to address the underlying vascular disease itself, by modifying and optimising vascular risk factors. Reducing further vascular damage can slow the rate of cognitive decline. It could certainly be argued that this is also relevant for other forms of dementia, as vascular disease is only going to exacerbate symptoms of these other conditions.

In practice, optimisation of vascular risk factors includes:

- Regular physical exercise
- Eating a healthy diet low in saturated fat
- Maintaining a healthy weight
- Ensuring that blood pressure is well controlled (through diet, exercise and antihypertensives)
- Ensuring that blood cholesterol is well controlled (through diet and perhaps statins)
- Ruling out or treating diabetes
- Reducing alcohol intake and stopping smoking.

In some cases, aspirin may be used, though evidence suggests that, despite this blood-thinning agent being helpful in reducing vascular disease in general, it may not reduce the risk of vascular dementia specifically. If there is evidence of narrowing of the carotid arteries (which can be determined using an ultrasound), a *carotid endarterectomy* may be considered. This is a surgical operation in which a small incision is made in the carotid artery (there is one on either side of the neck) and the cause of the narrowing – normally an area of plaque created by a build-up of cholesterol and calcium – is removed.

Dementia with Lewy bodies and Parkinson's disease

These two conditions, which share a similar underlying pathology (see Chapter 9), are considered by many to have more of a deficit of acetylcholine than that seen in Alzheimer's disease, and one could therefore predict that cholinesterase inhibitors may be of benefit. The evidence of effectiveness from studies, however, is mixed.

My experience is that both conditions can respond favourably to cholinesterase inhibitors, in regard to cognitive symptoms as well as behavioural and psychological symptoms. On the whole, the drugs seem to be well tolerated.

Studies looking at the role of memantine in treating these conditions are generally favourable, though are considered to be of low quality. It is hard to draw firm conclusions about the medication's use in these conditions.

Frontotemporal dementia

Unfortunately, there is no compelling evidence to support the use of cholinesterase inhibitors or memantine in frontotemporal dementia when attempting to preserve cognitive function. Additionally, cholinesterase inhibitors can worsen behavioural symptoms in frontotemporal dementia.

Alcohol-related dementia

Although there are a few small studies showing that both memantine and one of the cholinesterase inhibitors (rivastigmine) may provide cognitive benefit in alcohol-related dementia, these findings need to be replicated before we can feel confident that either style of medication has a role to play in treating this condition

The most important treatment in alcohol-related dementia is for the patient to stop drinking alcohol. As we saw in Chapter 9, this may even reverse some cognitive deficits. With enduring abstinence, improvements may continue over a period of months.

Replacement of vitamins, especially B1 and thiamine, may also help preserve cognition, while general improvements in lifestyle – regular exercise and healthy eating – may also be of benefit. Treating other diseases that may contribute to cognitive loss (such as obesity and vascular disease) is also important.

Other dementias

Neither AIDS dementia complex (ADC) nor Huntington's dementia have been sufficiently studied to assess the effectiveness of cholinesterase inhibitors or memantine. There is also insufficient evidence to recommend the routine use of cholinesterase inhibitors in other, rarer forms of dementia.

16

Behavioural and Psychological Symptoms of Dementia

- Behavioural and psychological symptoms of dementia (BPSD) are very common, and can be a cause of considerable distress to the individual with the condition and those around them. They are often an attempt to communicate an unmet need such as pain, fear, boredom or loneliness.

- There are multiple models of BPSD, which are not mutually exclusive. These models often recognise the individuality of the person and the need to respect and understand their own personal experiences.

- Non-drug measures should always be tried first in the management of BPSD – unless there is an immediate risk of harm to the person or others, or high levels of individual distress.

- Medications can sometimes make a significant difference to the quality of life of the person for whom they are prescribed, as well as for those around them.

- A cautious approach to the use of medication is critical: starting at a low dose, recognising individual vulnerabilities to side effects, closely monitoring for improvements, being mindful of side effects and ceasing the medication if it is unhelpful.

- BPSD may improve spontaneously even though the dementia gets worse.

- Physical and chemical restraint is rarely necessary and can result in significant harm.

In this chapter we will discuss one of the most distressing and difficult aspects of dementia: the *behavioural and psychological symptoms of dementia* (BPSD), a term that encompasses a large number of non-cognitive symptoms associated with the condition.

In my experience, BPSD often cause carers much more concern and anguish than the cognitive symptoms of dementia and are frequently the reason that a carer feels compelled to place their loved one in an aged-care facility. Unfortunately, they are also very common: a large majority of those with dementia will experience at least one symptom during the course of their illness. Prompt recognition and effective treatment can delay the need for this placement and allow the individual experiencing dementia to stay in their own home for longer. Recognising their presence, and knowing that difficult and confronting behaviours are related to the underlying disease rather than to the person, often helps those around them cope with their ramifications. For this reason, I will go into some detail about the nature of BPSD, and what can be done to treat them.

What are BPSD?

BPSD have been defined as 'symptoms of disturbed perception, thought content, mood or behaviour that frequently occur in patients with dementia'. The *behavioural* manifestations, which are usually based on observation of the individual with dementia, include:

- Physical aggression
- Apathy
- Sleep disturbance
- Loud vocalisations (including screaming)
- Sexually disinhibited behaviour
- Restlessness and agitation
- Wandering
- Hoarding
- Shadowing (following care staff or relatives around constantly).

The *psychological* symptoms include:

- Changes in mood (such as depression)
- Anxiety
- Psychotic symptoms (including delusions, hallucinations and misidentification)
- Irritability
- Emotional lability (the inability to control one's emotional state).

Unfortunately, most individuals with dementia will encounter these difficult symptoms at some point in the illness. Mood symptoms commonly occur in the early stages of the illness, while agitation and psychotic behaviours are more frequent in the moderate stage. Many BPSD may spontaneously settle as the dementia progresses. Their impact may also be lessened as time goes by, in part due to the deteriorating physical and neurological abilities. For example, the individual may be too weak for aggression to be problematic.

Studies looking at the types and rates of BPSD in different types of dementia have demonstrated mixed results. Some have shown little difference between vascular dementia and Alzheimer's disease, while others have shown increased rates of depression in vascular dementia and higher rates of delusions in Alzheimer's disease.

It is generally considered that depression, emotional lability and apathy are strongly associated with vascular dementia, and that mixed dementia seems to produce the highest level of psychiatric disturbance. Visual hallucinations are more common in dementia with Lewy bodies (occurring in 80 per cent of cases) than in Alzheimer's disease (20 per cent of cases). Frontotemporal dementia is associated with higher levels of numerous behavioural symptoms, including impulsivity, compulsive behaviours, hypersexuality and verbal outbursts. Huntington's disease dementia has been associated with the early appearance of disruptive and difficult behaviours; these may precede cognitive symptoms.

Specific BPSD

Owing to different study designs, the rates of individual BPSD in those with dementia tends to vary considerably, though some are certainly more common than others. Let's look at some of these symptoms in more detail.

Delusions

Delusions are false *beliefs* that are held firmly, and that are immune to counterargument. The frequency with which they occur is cited as being between 10 and 73 per cent. In the context of dementia, delusions take a number of common forms:

- *A belief that people are stealing things.* This often follows the individual forgetting where they have put something and, after being unable to locate it, assuming it must have been stolen.
- *A belief that a house is not one's home.* Despite residing in a nursing home for many years, an individual may believe they have to return home; this may lead to problematic wandering.
- *A belief that a spouse is an imposter.* This is also known as a Capgras delusion; naturally, it can be very distressing for both parties.
- *A belief of being unduly abandoned by family.* This occurs especially after being placed in supported care.
- *A belief that a partner is being unfaithful.*

Predictably, delusions can lead to considerable distress, which sometimes presents as verbal or physical aggression. It is important to note that, by definition, you will not be able to convince someone with a delusion that their thinking is faulty. It is important to recognise this, as trying to do so may aggravate the person and affect the trust you have with them. Acknowledgement of their distress (which *is* real) and gentle redirection to other topics is a preferred response.

Hallucinations

A hallucination is a false *perception*. The person experiencing a hallucination senses that someone (or something) is present when there is nothing there. Hallucinations can occur in any sensory modality (vision, hearing, touch or smell), and affect roughly 10–50 per cent of those with dementia.

In dementia, visual hallucinations are most common (especially in dementia with Lewy bodies), though auditory hallucinations are not infrequent. Other sensory hallucinations (such as of touch or smell) are rare. A specific visual hallucination in dementia seems to be that of imagining people (strangers or family) to be in the home (so-called *phantom boarders*). As with delusions, hallucinations can be a source of significant distress.

It should be noted that sensory deficits (hearing and visual problems) can increase the risk of hallucinations, so addressing these represents an important potential aspect of treatment.

Misidentification

These are also disorders of perception, though they differ from hallucinations in that they are based on something or someone that *is* present but that is misrecognised. These may include:

- Misidentifying oneself, such as in a mirror; this is known as the *mirror sign*
- Misidentifying people in one's own home; this is known as the *phantom boarder sign* (see above; the phantom boarder phenomenon can also occur as a hallucination)
- Misidentifying other people
- Misconstruing events on TV as occurring in the immediate environment.

Apathy

Often confused with depression, which can present with a similar picture of inertia, apathy is a state of impaired motivation and disinterest that leads to inactivity. It is very common in dementia, and is identifiable by a lack of social interaction, initiative, enthusiasm and emotional responsiveness.

Unlike depression, apathy does not usually produce evidence of depressed mood, negative thinking, tearfulness or thoughts of suicide, or disturbance of sleep or appetite. The individual may not appear distressed in themselves, and may not see any problem with their lack of initiative. Apathy can be a major challenge for a carer, however, who may constantly feel the need to encourage their loved one to do anything, including self-care.

Anxiety

In my experience, anxiety is common and tends to be more severe in mild and moderate dementia, reducing as the dementia progresses. Much of the anxiety is understandable as a concern about diminishing control over one's affairs and the inevitable future cognitive losses. Loss of executive function – a skill that allows us to rationalise problems – may also lead to increased anxiety.

People may experience specific anxieties over affairs that were once not of concern – chiefly finances, the future and one's health. Anxiety may also be a phenomenon secondary to other BPSD, such as delusional beliefs about being abandoned.

A specific anxiety about an upcoming event may result in *Godot syndrome*, where the individual repeatedly asks for details, to the point where it becomes distressing and burdensome for the carer. Another specific fear – that of being left alone or abandoned – can also be very difficult for a carer to manage. It can result in the anxious individual shadowing the carer wherever they go, even if it is just into another room.

Individuals with anxiety may seem restless, agitated and fretful, and sometimes anxiety may lead to aggression as the person struggles to comprehend what others are doing for them. Trouble getting to sleep may be a problem, as may a reduction in appetite.

Depression

Periods of depressed mood are very common in dementia. A significant proportion of individuals have symptoms either of a *major depressive disorder* or of *sub-syndromal depression*. Having experienced depression before the onset of dementia increases the likelihood of this occurring.

Interviewing someone in the early stages of dementia who also has depression will reveal symptoms of the mood disorder similar to those seen in people without dementia. They may describe low mood, negative thinking, lack of enjoyment and even, if the depression is severe, thoughts that they may be better off dead. As the dementia progresses, however, many of the symptoms of depression (such as apathy, weight loss, lack of interest, sleep disturbance or agitation) may equally be due to the underlying dementia. Coupled with this, language function often deteriorates with dementia, and verbal responses to questions asked about depression may not be reliable.

There are, however, certain red flags that may indicate the presence of depression in someone with dementia. These include:

- Acute and inexplicable behaviour changes
- Consistently low mood and loss of pleasure
- Family suspicion of depression
- Self-deprecatory statements and expressions of a desire to die
- A past history or family history of depression
- A rapid decline in cognition.

Sudden unexpected episodes of tearfulness, although possibly a sign of depression, should not be assumed to be so: they may equally be due to the loss of emotional control that can accompany dementia. In this case, the crying often is incongruous with what is going on around the person at the time – that is, there may be nothing to explain why the crying is occurring. This is known as *emotional lability*.

In evaluating depression in dementia, a measure called the *Cornell scale* can be quite helpful.

Wandering

Wandering behaviour may include aimless walking and exit-seeking behaviours. Safe wandering is not necessarily a bad thing, but wandering is often a manifestation of another psychological problem, such as anxiety, boredom or paranoia. It may also be related to the disoriented state of the individual. Wandering can be quite troublesome for carers, and the attendant risks – such as the person leaving the house and getting lost, or falling over – are commonly the reason for placing someone with dementia in residential care. Wandering can occur during the day or at night. GPS bracelets, personal identity documents (perhaps on a lanyard or in a wallet) and personal alarms can all be helpful. Keeping 'triggers' for exit-seeking (such as keys or coats) out of sight may also help. Recognising the various reasons why someone might want to leave the place where they are can be helpful in addressing the behaviour. The person may be following an old routine (believing they are off to work, for instance), or trying to get to the toilet, or fearful of where they are. Wandering can be secondary to an *unmet need*, detailed later in this chapter.

Agitation and aggression

Agitation is defined as 'inappropriate verbal, vocal or motor activity that is not judged by an observer to result directly from the needs or confusion of the person'. There may be numerous influencing factors, including the direct neurobiological effects of the underlying dementia, psychological factors (such as depression, anxiety or psychosis), other medical factors (such as pain, breathlessness or constipation), social and environmental factors, and aspects of the person's underlying personality.

Four subtypes of agitation have been recognised:

- *Physically non-aggressive behaviours.* These include restlessness, hyperactivity, repetitiveness, wandering, rummaging and pacing.
- *Physically aggressive behaviours.*
- *Verbally non-aggressive behaviours.* These include requests for attention, bossiness, complaining, repetitive questions and anxious complaints.
- *Verbally aggressive behaviours.* Examples include screaming and cursing.

General strategies to address aggression include remaining calm but vigilant about potential risk, and maintaining a safe distance (so it is easy to move out of harm's way, but also so as not to be seen as threatening). Using a measured and not overly loud voice and avoiding entering arguments are also advised. Sometimes, if there is no immediate danger, moving away and allowing the person space can be very helpful.

Resistiveness to care

This type of BPSD is specific in its presentation, pertaining only to times when care (such as attendance to personal hygiene) is being provided. It is positively correlated with the severity of the cognitive impairment, as well as with loss of insight. It may be passive or active, and associated with verbal or physical aggression. Like many of the other BPSD, it is understandable, especially given the intimate nature of the care that often needs to be given. It may occur secondarily to other BPSD, such as anxiety, apathy or paranoid delusions.

Sexual disinhibition

This term refers to inappropriate sexualised verbal and physical behaviours. Examples include sexualised remarks aimed at care staff, inappropriate touching and public masturbation. Such behaviours can be very troublesome for carers, both in a home environment and in residential care. They can pose difficult ethical dilemmas related to interpretation of normal sexual behaviour. See Chapter 18 for a further exploration of this topic.

Disruptive vocalising

Also referred to as 'calling out' or vocally disruptive behaviour, this is a not uncommon problem in dementia. It is often a manifestation of another type of BPSD, occurring for instance as a consequence of anxiety or in response to hallucinations, and can be one of the more difficult conditions to treat. It may also occur as a consequence of understimulation (boredom and social isolation) or overstimulation (such as too much noise). Physical health conditions, especially pain, may also underpin disruptive vocalising.

Vocalising may be quiet – taking the form of moaning or murmuring – and may therefore be overlooked. If it is missed this can be a problem, especially if it's a sign of some other problem.

It is much more likely to be noticed when it is high-volume and causing distress or disturbance to others. Screaming is an extreme form of vocalising, and may occur day or night. Often it is difficult to understand the content of what is being said, though there is frequently a repetitive quality. Sometimes it may be a method of self-soothing.

Sleep disturbance

This is very common in dementia, and is sometimes associated with a reversal of *circadian rhythm*, meaning that large parts of the day are spent asleep and much of the night is spent awake. If the individual is being cared for at home, this can contribute greatly to caregiver distress, especially as it may lead to sleep deprivation for the carer themselves. See Chapter 17 for more on this.

A note on 'sundowning'

There may be significant fluctuations in the severity of BPSD from day to day and even from hour to hour. *Sundowning* is a classic example of this, and a term with which many involved in dementia care are familiar. It relates to the observation that BPSD commonly arise later in the day – as the sun goes down. This is especially the case in Alzheimer's disease, though it can occur in other dementias.

BPSD in residential care

It is worth mentioning the complexity that arises when an individual enters residential care. In my experience, BPSD are a common cause of friction between the staff involved in the day-to-day care of the individual with dementia and the relatives who come to visit. A number of factors contribute to this, including the inadequate staffing levels at most aged-care facilities – meaning that the optimal scenario of one-to-one care, as may have occurred at home, is no longer possible. This may lead to distress on the part of relatives who worry that their loved one is not receiving adequate attention.

The priorities and concerns of relatives and care staff may also differ. The primary focus of a relative is, quite rightly, the safety and welfare of their loved one. Although this should be of paramount importance to care staff also, they must balance the needs of that individual with the needs and rights of other residents, as well as with their own needs and rights in their workplace.

Staff may have to deal with difficult behaviours that are not apparent to relatives. In my experience, when relatives visit BPSD are far less evident or problematic, which means relatives may not fully appreciate their severity or frequency. This temporary quiescence of BPSD may in part be due to the emotional connection that exists between the patient and their relative, and the fact they are receiving one-to-one attention. Because they see their loved one 'at their best', it can be hard for the relative to believe staff reports that their loved one has been physically aggressive or very distressed.

Relatives often also visit at times not classically associated with triggers for BPSD – for example, when care such as showering or dressing need to be provided. Sometimes relatives confide in me that they feel the problem is how staff approach their loved one. Although this can be the cause, often it is not. In my experience, almost all staff are trying to do their best in a difficult situation, and BPSD may persist despite them making substantial and appropriate changes to how they manage things.

The type of BPSD that most commonly causes this tension is physical aggression. Unfortunately, despite the best efforts of staff, an aggression risk sometimes escalates to the point where there is a danger of someone (another resident or a member of staff) becoming seriously harmed, and the only intervention that is likely to be effective is one that involves medication. These medications can cause side effects, however, which may increase the risk of harm to the individual receiving them; if they are over-sedated, for instance, this can cause them to fall.

What, then, is the answer? It really depends on priorities, and if these differ in the minds of the various people involved in the care of someone with dementia, then a solution can be hard to find. I am regularly involved in such dilemmas in my clinical work as a psychogeriatrician, and I think the answer lies partly in the ability of all parties involved to have a frank and open-minded discussion about risk. This requires diplomacy, actively listening to all the different points of view, and the provision of enough clinical information for everyone to make an informed decision.

Clearly, too, there needs to be clear documentation of incidents that have occurred and their contexts, and what has been done to address them. Usually I find that once family members are satisfied that all non-drug measures have been considered and/or tried, they are more amenable to considering the need for medication, at least in the short term, and this can sometimes be of great benefit.

Treatments for BPSD

Non-drug treatments

It is universally accepted that if problems can be addressed without the need for medication, that is preferable. In this way, any side effects are minimised – something that is especially important for an individual experiencing dementia, who may be physically frail and whose brain may be particularly vulnerable to the effects of any medication. In recognition of this, the emphasis when treating BPSD should be on non-pharmacological methods, at least in the first instance. The only exception is when there is an acute risk of the individual hurting themselves or someone else, either deliberately or through misadventure.

A number of models have been put forward to explain BPSD, including:

- The 'unmet needs' model
- The behavioural model
- The biological model
- The theory of reduced stress threshold in dementia.

These models are not mutually exclusive, and different symptoms may be explained in various ways. The models are helpful, however, in allowing us to understand BPSD and create strategies to manage them.

The unmet needs model

One useful approach to BPSD is to consider them through the prism of *unmet needs*. That is to say, the behaviour or psychological disturbance is an articulation of a problem that cannot otherwise be expressed. The unmet needs model proposes that problem behaviours are a complex phenomenon affected by an interaction of cognitive impairment, physical health, mental health, past habits and personality, and environmental factors. It also presupposes that the person experiencing BPSD is unable to communicate what their concerns may be.

Central to the concept of unmet needs is the requirement to *know* the person who has dementia. Only in this way can we get an adequate understanding of what might be done to help them. This knowledge should include the following:

- Their underlying personality:
  ○ Do they enjoy the company of others or does it make them anxious?
  ○ Do they enjoy noise and activity or do they prefer peace and quiet? It should be noted that dementia often causes difficulties in filtering out or ignoring the various things going on in our environment, meaning that if there is too much going on then it can cause distress.
  ○ What fears do they have?
  ○ What traumas have they suffered over their lives? Has lack of money been a problem? Have they been abused in some way (meaning that physical closeness may be more threatening)? Have they been abandoned as a youngster, or left by a spouse, feeding into a fear of being left alone?
  ○ How would they normally cope with stress? What are the usual signs? Some people withdraw and others get angry.
  ○ Do they have certain racial prejudices?
  ○ What have they enjoyed doing over their lives? What were their hobbies?
  ○ What have they disliked?
  ○ What has been their line of work? Could that explain their repetitive behaviours?

- Their capacity to articulate their concerns and understand what is happening:
  - Do they have expressive dysphasia, which prevents them from communicating their needs?
  - Do they have receptive dysphasia, meaning they do not understand what is being said to them or asked of them?
  - Do they speak the same language as those around them? This is not a problem particular to dementia, of course, though translation issues may be exacerbated in this condition.
- Their physical health:
  - Are they in pain?
  - Are they constipated?
  - Might they have a urinary tract infection?
  - Are they unable to pass urine?
  - Are they tired?
  - Could their medications be causing side effects?
  - Can they hear properly?
  - Can they see properly?
  - Are they hungry?
  - Are they thirsty?
- Their psychological health:
  - Are they bored?
  - Are they lonely?
  - Are they depressed?
  - Are they anxious?
  - Are they fearful?
  - Are they frustrated by their incapacity?
  - Are they responding to a hallucination or delusion?
- Their physical and social environment:
  - Is it too noisy? Too quiet?
  - Is the environment easy to navigate?
  - Is there enough to do?
  - Is the temperature okay?
  - Are they physically comfortable? Would they prefer to be in a chair or in bed?
  - Do they have somewhere they can be in peace, away from others?

  ° Are there others around them who are causing them
    distress?
  ° Are the caregivers empathic and patient? Do they explain
    what they are doing as they are doing it?
  ° What are their specific cultural or religious needs?
  ° Are they being offered food they like or are used to? Is it
    culturally appropriate?
  ° What is their sexual orientation? Is this a factor in the
    presenting behaviour?

These questions emphasise the optimal approach to BPSD management: *patient-centred care.* This recognises the individuality of the person with dementia. It also allows for a thorough and comprehensive analysis of the problem in order to identify issues that may not otherwise be picked up. Using this model, we can correct issues in the various domains, whether they involve physical health problems, psychosocial triggers or environmental concerns.

The behavioural model

This model can be very useful in determining the cause of the BPSD and how to remedy it. It incorporates the idea of a sequence of events – the antecedent, the behaviour and the consequence (ABC) – underpinning the BPSD.

The *antecedent* is the trigger for the *behaviour*, which then results in a *consequence*. By using this model we can examine what in the environment might have caused the behaviour, and whether the consequences of the behaviour are likely to reinforce it or deter it in the future.

Let's consider an example. Perhaps an individual becomes agitated whenever there is too much noise in the environment (the antecedent). Lessening the exposure to the noise (either by reducing the noise or taking the individual somewhere quiet) may help settle the behaviour. Alternatively, if the consequence of a person being disruptive is to provide them with something they like to eat or to give them craved-for one-to-one attention, this may inadvertently reinforce the behaviour.

To optimise the chances of success, it is important that people who know the patient well – usually family members – are involved in developing a plan. This is especially relevant when the individual is in residential care, where the staff, at least initially, may know very little about the person's background.

The biological model

This model assumes that behaviours are essentially a consequence of neurological changes in the brain, and therefore are a direct symptom of the disease process. One advantage of this approach is that it acknowledges that not all behaviours are understandable on the basis of the unmet needs model or the behavioural model, and therefore a lack of success in optimising these variables is not a reflection of failure by the caregiver (believing otherwise does little but increase carer stress).

This biological approach also allows us to think of possible pharmacological interventions, targeting the neurobiological abnormalities we know to be associated with dementia. (We'll discuss these interventions later in this chapter.)

The progressively lowered stress threshold model

This model considers that the capacity of an individual to deal with stress becomes increasingly impaired as the brain becomes progressively more damaged. Stress inducers include physical stressors (such as pain or infection), misleading stimuli or inappropriate stimuli, a change of environment, caregiver or routine, an internal or external demand that exceeds functional capacity, fatigue, and the affective (mood-related) response to perceptions of loss.

This approach may explain why agitation often becomes progressively worse as the day goes on – due to accumulation of stressors over this time. A number of helpful interventions may arise as a result. We can:

- Maximise safe function by supporting losses in a prosthetic manner (such as by using a wheelie walker if there are problems with mobility)
- Provide unconditional positive regard

- Use the patient's anxiety and agitation as an indicator of their activity and stimulation level
- Teach caregivers to observe and 'listen' to patients
- Modify environments to support losses and enhance safety
- Provide ongoing support for informal and formal caregivers.

Specific non-medication measures

One of the difficulties in studying how well non-drug measures work in treating BPSD is that there is usually a common ingredient of positive human interaction which itself may improve BPSD. Evidence suggests that the following specific interventions are helpful in BPSD, however:

- *Psychoeducation for patients and caregivers.* This involves the provision of information about the problems faced, such as that given above. The more you know about a problem, the greater your chances of finding a solution. Practically, this might involve reading up on BPSD or attending workshops or sessions on the topic. (These are often run by local support groups or carers groups – see the Appendix for further information.) For care staff in residential care, this may involve in-house or external training.
- *Physical exercise.* Regular physical activity (as long as it does not provoke pain) can help reduce BPSD.
- *Sensory stimulation.* Use of a *Snoezelen room* (a space that provides soothing multisensory stimuli), for example, is known to be effective at reducing agitation and disruptive behaviour, though the effects are short term, occurring mainly during the treatment and for a short time afterwards.
- *Music therapy.* This likewise may be helpful for the time it is being employed.
- *Reality orientation therapy.* This is therapy that helps us know better where we are in time and space, and it can be of some benefit.
- *Reminiscence therapy.* Using objects from everyday life to stimulate memory – photos, for example – seems to improve mood in those with dementia.
- *Cognitive behavioural therapy* (CBT). These techniques seem to

benefit anxiety, aggression and agitation in dementia and the effects appear to last some months. This is best for those in the mild to moderate stages of the disease. CBT involves looking at the way the mind works when we are stressed, depressed or angry and challenging ourselves to change these unhelpful ways of thinking. It may also investigate how our behaviours may be influencing our feelings; for example, staying in bed all day, despite being what we may want to do, is unlikely to help us overcome the feeling of depression. CBT encourages us to engage in more adaptive (helpful) behaviours.

- *Aromatherapy.* There is modest evidence that aromatherapy, particularly with lavender oils, may reduce agitation.

Another intervention that has some evidence of effectiveness is *doll therapy*. This involves giving an individual with (advanced) dementia a lifelike doll that they can care for and love. There is considerable anecdotal evidence that this can be soothing for some, and can bring back happy memories from years before, though it is not without controversy – some opponents believe it is demeaning. This is, of course, a matter of personal judgement, and perhaps there is no right or wrong. My experience is that it can be very helpful for certain individuals in reducing agitation.

Pet therapy (or *animal-assisted therapy*) is another treatment that is commonly used, and recognises that loneliness and boredom, which may contribute to BPSD, can be eased by the presence of animals. Again, much of the evidence is anecdotal, though there have been a few formal studies to support its use.

Carer approach and BPSD

The approach of the carer is of critical importance, and can make a very significant difference to the nature and severity of BPSD. The following carer behaviours are unhelpful and likely to *increase* BPSD:

- Making sudden changes in the individual's environment or routine
- Imposing unrealistic demands

- Expressing negative emotions such as anger or aggression
- Being overly controlling or inflexible
- Being critical
- Repeatedly prompting individuals, with the hope that they will eventually remember or do something
- Belittling or talking down to them, or ignoring them.

Some of the more unhelpful carer approaches to BPSD occur as a consequence of carer stress. It is therefore important that this is recognised and addressed (see Chapter 23).

On the other hand, some caregiver behaviours can *reduce* BPSD. These include:

- Being warm, affectionate and empathic in all approaches
- Being flexible and adaptable and retaining a sense of humour
- Having a realistic appraisal of the person's capabilities
- Fostering their strengths
- Respecting that the individual still has valid emotions and feelings
- Being open to discussing the concerns of others and fostering a support network.

In Australia, we have access to a government-funded service that can provide advice to family carers, as well as to staff at residential facilities, about non-pharmacological approaches to BPSD. Known as Dementia Support Australia (DSA), this organisation provides two particularly helpful services: the Dementia Behaviour Management Advisory Service (DBMAS) and the Severe Behavioural Response Team (SBRT).

The DBMAS provides home visits in the community, and they also visit aged-care facilities. The SBRT provide a home visit service to aged-care facilities. Importantly, carers can refer their loved ones to be seen by one of these services. I have found their involvement to be invaluable. Their website also provides lots of advice about managing different aspects of dementia. Their publication entitled *A Guide for Family Carers: Dealing with behaviours in people with dementia* is a great resource for anyone who wants to know more about BPSD. (See the Appendix for further details.)

Treatments involving medication

In an ideal world, there would be no need for medications in the treatment of BPSD. Such a place would be populated by carers who have an infinite capacity to cope and who are invulnerable to verbal and physical abuse. They would not need to sleep or have time to themselves and there would always be a practical behavioural or environmental strategy to solve the problem at hand. In this world, there would also be no need to consider the welfare of other individuals with dementia or physical frailty living in close proximity, and there would exist the capacity to provide, at any given minute, one-to-one care.

Of course, that is not the world we live in. In the real world, carers are vulnerable, patients are often highly distressed despite the best efforts of their carers to solve problems through psychosocial means, and staffing levels at aged-care facilities are woefully inadequate. For this reason, in my opinion, there is a role for medications in the treatment of BPSD – especially when non-drug measures have not worked and/or there are high levels of distress or risk associated with the BPSD.

A recent Australian study of over 300,000 people, 50 per cent of whom had a diagnosis of dementia, revealed some sobering findings. In particular, the rate of use of antipsychotic medications doubled in the three months before entry into residential care, and then doubled again in the three months after entering residential care. Although not as dramatic, there were increases in the use of benzodiazepines and antidepressants as well. Many of these medications continued to be used for some time after the initial three months, which is also of potential concern.

Of course, there may have been good reasons for some of the increased prescribing. Increasing carer stress at home related to BPSD may have resulted in the use of these medications and then the need for placement. Also, the transition period as an individual with dementia enters care is often difficult, meaning that BPSD may be exacerbated for some weeks to months. Nonetheless, the study draws attention to a potentially worrying trend – not only that there may be over-prescription in the first place, but also that there is inadequate deprescribing (taking someone off a medication) when they are settled.

The principles of using medications

Any consideration of treating BPSD with medication must include the following:

- Weighing up the potential benefits and risks associated with using the medication. Some individuals may be at higher risk of side effects from specific medications than others, and this is therefore a personalised assessment.
- Starting at a low dose of the medication, and increasing slowly, while monitoring for side effects. At the same time, too cautious an approach may lead to an individual being undertreated. Frequent reassessment is necessary.
- Ensuring that an adequate dose of the medication is used (if tolerated) for an adequate length of time before abandoning it.
- Regularly reviewing the need for the medication, acknowledging that many BPSD will spontaneously resolve with progression of the disease, and the needs of the person may change.
- Being aware that sometimes medications can make BPSD worse – for instance, by increasing confusion and disorientation, leading to increased anxiety.

The classes of medication commonly used to treat BPSD

There are a number of medications commonly used to treat BPSD if non-drug measures don't work, though most of the research has focused on Alzheimer's disease and vascular disease. The medications fall into the following categories:

- Antidepressant medications
- Mood stabilisers
- Benzodiazepines
- Antipsychotic medications
- Cholinesterase inhibitors
- Memantine.

Although many of the medications listed may have non-specific benefits, the best approach to selecting medications for BPSD involves trying to detect constellations of symptoms that may indicate a certain domain of psychological disturbance. Symptoms may be suggestive of a depressive condition, anxiety or psychosis. Medications can then be selected on the basis of their specific efficacy in addressing these types of symptoms. Depression, for instance, should be treated with antidepressants, whereas psychotic symptoms such as hallucinations and delusions are less likely to respond to this class of medication, and so antipsychotics may be required.

The presentation of the psychiatric illnesses may be different, and often muted, resulting in sub-syndromal symptoms when occurring in someone with dementia. The following symptoms, however, are suggestive of each of these different psychological syndromes:

- Depression may be evident through periods of tearfulness, poor appetite, loss of motivation, changes in sleep pattern, articulation of negative thinking, lack of interest and thoughts of being better off dead.
- Anxiety may be indicated by restlessness, pacing, repetitive questioning and reassurance seeking, as well as sleep disturbance. Individuals may be too restless to even eat. When distracted, however, they are more likely to react in a positive fashion than someone with depression.
- Psychosis is characterised by the presence of hallucinations and/or delusions.
   - *Hallucinations* occur when an individual imagines seeing something that is not there, or hearing something that is not there. Dementia itself can cause visual hallucinations, in particular. These can often be quite distressing and frightening.
   - *Delusions* are false beliefs which are impossible to challenge. They often take the form of paranoid ideas, such as that items are being stolen, food is being poisoned, or the person is being kept prisoner. It should be noted that psychotic symptoms that occur purely as a consequence of dementia rather than another psychotic illness (such as schizophrenia) tend to be a lot more understandable and less bizarre.

The response to psychiatric medications is often not immediate, and this poses a clinical challenge. It may take weeks to months for a new medication to exert its full effect (though less so for benzodiazepines), and one must be careful not to increase the dose too soon and thus induce side effects unnecessarily.

It is worthwhile discussing the common side effects of the medications employed for BPSD. In my discussions with relatives, there is often particular concern about the use of antipsychotics due to widely circulated reports about serious side effects. Although these findings are indisputable, selectively highlighting risk in this way can be problematic. First, such coverage of the problems associated with antipsychotics tends to overshadow the possible side effects of other medications, which can be equally problematic. Also, the awareness can cause such reluctance to use antipsychotics that they are not used at all, or their use is inappropriately delayed. This may mean an individual with dementia suffers unduly, remaining anguished for long periods by their paranoid delusions, or that the risk they pose to others remains unnecessarily high.

Let's therefore look at the indications and effectiveness of the various medications commonly used, as well as their side effects.

Antidepressants

There are a number of classes of antidepressants. The most common used in dementia, but also in general, are the *selective serotonin reuptake inhibitors* (SSRIs). Examples include citalopram, escitalopram, sertraline, escitalopram, paroxetine and fluoxetine (these are their generic names; there are multiple brand names of each). As their title suggests, they all selectively affect serotonin receptors in the brain. This neurotransmitter has been implicated in depression, anxiety and a number of other BPSD, including those underpinned by agitation, impulsivity, apathy and disinhibition. Use of an SSRI can therefore help with these concerns.

SSRIs may transiently increase anxiety when prescribed, though this normally settles down after a period of days. Other known side effects include an increased risk of falls as well as a risk of gastrointestinal bleeding. They can also induce confusion and may cause blood sodium levels to drop. This latter concern can cause very significant medical problems, and may even, if severe and untreated, lead to seizures and death. It is, however, easily monitored through blood tests. It is generally recommended that individuals have their sodium level checked before commencement, shortly after starting and then periodically while on the medication.

Some SSRIs in high doses – particularly citalopram – can cause an abnormality of heart rhythm (QTc prolongation) that can be serious. Again, this can be monitored relatively easily by obtaining an ECG.

Mirtazapine, which also increases serotonin (by a different mechanism to the SSRIs), as well as increasing noradrenaline, another neurotransmitter, is also sometimes used. Mirtazapine can be particularly helpful to manage anxiety as well as low mood, especially when there is associated insomnia. Its chief side effects include sedation (it is given at night to enhance sleep, and sometimes the soporific effect can carry over to the next morning; this usually eases with time) and weight gain. It may also cause ankle swelling and some individuals report nightmares. Mirtazapine can also cause low sodium, though probably not as readily as SSRIs.

Other dual-acting antidepressants, which also affect serotonin and noradrenaline levels (such as venlafaxine, desvenlafaxine and duloxetine), can sometimes be helpful. These often have a more potent antidepressant effect, and have a side effect profile similar to that of SSRIs, though they also can cause high blood pressure, particularly at higher doses.

Tricyclic antidepressants (such as nortriptyline, amitriptyline, clomipramine and dothiepin), although very helpful for cognitively intact individuals experiencing depression or anxiety, are best not used first line in dementia due to their cognitive and other problematic side effects. Occasional low doses may be helpful for sleep and can be well tolerated.

Trazadone is an antidepressant that is unavailable in Australia, though it does have some evidence of effectiveness in BPSD, especially depression, anxiety, agitation and insomnia. It also affects serotonin levels and its chief side effects include sedation and postural hypotension (abnormal lowering of blood pressure when getting up). It is a rare cause also of priapism, a condition in which penile erections are pathologically prolonged.

In general, antidepressants may be particularly effective when depressive features, or features of anxiety, are prominent. They can also be used to treat agitation, apathy, disruptive vocalisations and sexually disinhibited behaviours. There is even evidence that one SSRI, citalopram, can treat psychotic symptoms.

Antidepressants may be especially helpful for reducing behavioural disturbance in some with frontotemporal dementia.

Drug	Starting dose (mg)	Dose range (mg) schedule
Trazadone	25	50–300
Citalopram	10	10–40
Escitalopram	5	10–20
Sertraline	25	50–100
Venlafaxine	37.5	75–150
Mirtazapine	15★	15–45
Duloxetine	30	30–60

★ I sometimes start at 7.5mg if insomnia is the main concern.

Dosing schedule for selected antidepressants in patients with dementia.

Adapted from IPA Complete Guides to Behavioral and Psychological Symptoms of Dementia (BPSD).

Mood stabilisers

The two most commonly used mood stabilisers are sodium valproate and carbamazepine. Both were originally used for treatment of epilepsy but are now used for a number of other conditions, including BPSD.

The evidence for *carbamazepine* being helpful for BPSD comes from only two small studies, which showed it may be helpful in quelling agitation, aggression and hostility. Ultimate dose ranges used in these studies were between 300 milligrams and 400 milligrams per day. It should be noted that these studies only looked at treatment over a number of weeks.

Carbamazepine may cause sedation and confusion, related to the dose used. It may also rarely cause a disorder called Stevens–Johnson syndrome, the most obvious manifestation of which is a rash. This needs to be closely monitored while the medication is prescribed. Carbamazepine may also cause liver damage and changes in the constituents of blood. My experience of carbamazepine suggests it can be helpful for some, especially if there are tolerability concerns with other medications.

The evidence for *sodium valproate* is less compelling. It can be sedating, cause weight gain, induce tremor and cause changes in gait. It may also induce changes in liver function and its use mandates regular blood tests to check this. I have on occasion prescribed this medication – especially in liquid form when compliance with tablets is problematic, and where there appears to be prominent mood swings – but have found the results to be mixed.

Benzodiazepines

Benzodiazepines are used to manage agitation and anxiety, along with aggression. Examples include alprazolam, clonazepam, lorazepam, diazepam and oxazepam (again, these are generic names). Short-acting agents (such as temazepam and nitrazepam) may be used for sleep. They can be very effective, though side effects include increased confusion, sedation and falls. There is also a concern about tolerance (that is, the need to increase doses to achieve the same effect) and dependence (a reliance on the medication that results in a state of withdrawal when it is ceased). This means that if the individual has been on a benzodiazepine consistently for a number of weeks, any attempt to withdraw the medication should be done gradually. It also underpins the importance of using this style of medication for as short a period as possible.

One benefit of this style of medications is that they begin to work very rapidly (unlike, for instance, antidepressants, which may take weeks to be therapeutic). As with all medications, benzodiazepines should be used for as short a period as possible.

Benzodiazepine	Daily dose range (mg)*
Oxazepam	3.75 to 45
Diazepam	2 to 10
Lorazcpam	0.5 to 2
Temazepam	5 to 20 (at night)
Nitrazepam	2.5 to 5 (at night)

* Doses may be higher depending on response to medication.
Commonly prescribed benzodiazepine doses in the elderly.

Antipsychotics

Examples of this style of medication include risperidone, quetiapine, aripiprazole, olanzapine, lurasidone, paliperidone, amisulpride, ziprasidone and haloperidol.

Antipsychotic medications have received some bad press over the last decade. The inappropriate use of these, along with benzodiazepines, has recently been highlighted in Australia by the Royal Commission into Aged Care Quality and Safety, with a particular concern that they are being used simply as a chemical restraint. This attention is a welcome development, although there is now a risk that individuals may be undertreated, as relatives and medical practitioners become afraid to use antipsychotics. I have witnessed reluctance to use these drugs frequently over the years, and have sometimes regretted, after seeing a dramatic reduction in distress and risk with their use, that we had not started them earlier.

My opinion is that antipsychotics can be very helpful in certain cases, although the target symptoms must be clearly identified as responsive to this style of medication. It is generally considered that antipsychotics should be reserved for individuals in whom there are prominent psychotic features (hallucinations or delusions, including paranoia), a high risk of aggression, or high levels of agitation, and whose behaviours have been unresponsive to other medications. Generally, antipsychotics are not helpful for BPSD such as wandering, intrusive behaviours or disruptive vocalising, unless these are driven by a psychotic process.

Studies have demonstrated an increased risk of some serious medical problems developing with antipsychotics, regardless of which one is used (a so-called *class effect*). This includes an increased risk of cerebrovascular events (including stroke), heart attack or rhythm disturbance, and pneumonia. The risk of death from any cause also seems to be heightened with the use of these medications (about 1.6 times the risk, compared with placebo). The risk of side effects is correlated with the length of time individuals remain on the medication. Increased confusion can also occur as a class effect, and there is evidence that the cognitive decline seen in dementia may be accelerated with these medications. Additionally, there may be other negative effects, the risk of which is dependent to a degree on the choice of antipsychotic used. These are detailed below, but include sedation (potentially leading to falls, fractures, immobility and pressure areas, reduced oral intake and reduced social engagement) and parkinsonism. Metabolic syndrome – a constellation of symptoms including weight gain, elevated blood sugar and elevated blood fats – is also a well-known side effect of antipsychotics, and its development needs to be monitored.

A systematic review in 2016 demonstrated that the evidence for three atypical antipsychotics in treating BPSD (olanzapine, risperidone and aripiprazole) was greater than for certain others, such as quetiapine. This review also noted the paucity of data for a number of newer antipsychotics, such as lurasidone and paliperidone.

Risperidone can increase the risk of parkinsonism. This drug effect is so called due to the similar presentation to Parkinson's disease. Those with parkinsonism may develop increased tone in their muscles, as well as a tremor in their hands. They may find it hard to walk, to initiate movement or to rise from a chair. Their posture may become stooped. The risk of falls is increased. This side effect of parkinsonism is related to dose, however, and is not inevitable. It is also generally not permanent – that is, when the medication is removed, the parkinsonism should disappear. Complicating matters, the parkinsonism can be quite delayed in onset, perhaps not occurring for some weeks after the medication is introduced. Similarly, the parkinsonism may take some time to fully resolve after the medication has been ceased. To date, risperidone is the only antipsychotic that is licensed for use in Australia in treating BPSD.

Quetiapine is less likely to cause parkinsonism, and is my treatment of choice if antipsychotics are required for dementia in which this symptom commonly occurs, such as Parkinson's disease dementia or dementia with Lewy bodies. It may cause sedation and induce low blood pressure, however, which also increases the risk of falls. This is most noticeable as postural low blood pressure (that is, blood pressure that drops when moving from lying to sitting or from sitting to standing) and occurs particularly when the medication is first introduced or the dose increased. This medication can also induce weight gain and metabolic problems, though these issues do not appear to be too problematic in most of the elderly patients I have seen.

Olanzapine sits somewhere in the middle between quetiapine and risperidone in regard to the risk of parkinsonism. Similarly to quetiapine, it can induce weight gain and metabolic problems, and can also cause sedation. Swelling of the lower legs (peripheral oedema) may occur. At higher doses it can specifically impair cognition due to anticholinergic activity, and therefore has the potential to increase confusion.

Aripiprazole does not seem to carry the same risk as some other antipsychotics in regard to causing metabolic problems. For some it can be somewhat sedating, though for others it can seem to cause agitation and restlessness.

Haloperidol is an example of an older antipsychotic (known as *typical antipsychotics*, in contrast to the *atypical* agents such as risperidone, quetiapine and olanzapine). Typical agents have a higher propensity to cause parkinsonism than their atypical counterparts, but less in the way of metabolic disturbance.

Clozapine is a particularly effective antipsychotic used in many younger patients with treatment-refractory schizophrenia – that is, which has not responded to other antipsychotics. It has the advantage of causing minimal parkinsonism and therefore is theoretically a good choice for use in dementia due to Parkinson's disease or dementia with Lewy bodies. Unfortunately, however, it can cause a serious reduction in a type of white blood cell – causing impaired immunity – and its use mandates regular blood tests to monitor this. I have never used it for BPSD.

Other, newer antipsychotics such as amisulpride, lurasidone and ziprasidone do not have sufficient evidence to support their routine use in BPSD.

Drug	Starting dose (mg)	Dose range (mg) schedule
Risperidone	0.25	0.5–2 once daily
Olanzapine	2.5	5–10 once daily
Aripiprazole	2.0	5–10 daily
Quetiapine	25.0*	25–150 daily divided doses
Haloperidol	0.5	0.5–2 once daily

* I sometimes use 12.5mg initially

Clinical recommendations for dosing of typical and atypical antipsychotics for BPSD. Adapted from IPA Complete Guides to Behavioral and Psychological Symptoms of Dementia (BPSD).

If antipsychotic therapy is commenced, and the symptoms are well treated, it is best practice to try to withdraw the drug after a period of three months. This is in recognition of the fact that symptoms may spontaneously settle with progression of the dementia.

Cholinesterase inhibitors

Cholinesterase inhibitors include rivastigmine, donepezil and galantamine, and are detailed in Chapter 15 for their use as cognitive enhancers. They may play a role in treatment of BPSD, and for this reason they are sometimes used when the dementia is at a stage where there is unlikely to be much cognitive benefit. They may be helpful for a range of BPSD, including anxiety, depression, psychosis and agitation, and apathy. The effectiveness of this style of medication may be greater for delaying the onset of BPSD in the first place rather than for treating them when they are present.

These medications may, paradoxically, induce agitation (due to being a neuro-stimulant) and cause gastrointestinal symptoms, as well as exacerbating slow heart rate, gastric ulcer disease and restrictive lung disease. They may also increase the risk of falls. In my experience, however, they are reasonably well tolerated. The dosing of these style of medications for BPSD is the same as for cognitive enhancement, and is outlined in Chapter 15.

For both dementia with Lewy bodies and Parkinson's disease dementia, cholinesterase inhibitors are considered a good choice, especially given that individuals with these conditions may be particularly susceptible to side effects from antipsychotics. Cholinesterase inhibitors have the potential to worsen BPSD when used in those with frontotemporal dementia.

Memantine

Memantine, discussed in Chapter 15, seems to be especially effective when the dementia is at a moderate to severe phase. In my experience, it is reasonably well tolerated, though it can cause sedation, constipation, dizziness, high blood pressure, headaches and reduced appetite. Symptoms for which there is some evidence of response to memantine include irritability, psychosis, agitation and aggression, though the evidence overall is limited.

The dose of memantine for treating BPSD is the same as for treating cognitive problems: 20 milligrams per day. This is achieved by increasing the initial 5 milligram daily dose over a number of weeks. The response to memantine may therefore be somewhat delayed.

Medicinal cannabis

Cannabis, also known as marijuana, is derived from a plant called *Cannabis sativa*. This plant contains various chemicals known as *cannabinoids*. There are over 100 types of cannabinoid, though *tetrahydrocannabinol* (THC) is probably the one that people most associate with recreational use. This is the so-called *psychoactive* component, causing changes in mood and perception that we associate with being 'high'. The other dominant cannabinoid is *cannabidiol* (CBD), which lacks these psychoactive elements.

With the decriminalisation of cannabis for recreational use, and its legalisation in various parts of the world for medical purposes, there is increasing interest in its potential use in dementia.

Although cannabinoids may have neuroprotective effects – reducing neuroinflammation or ameliorating the damage caused by beta-amyloid and tau, for instance – cannabis is not currently used as a cognitive enhancement therapy in those with dementia.

The role of cannabis in treating BPSD has also not been studied extensively, though it is an area of increasing interest. Studies completed thus far have used THC, CBD and a combination of the two. One small Swiss study demonstrated considerable improvements in BPSD with the use of a combination of THC and CBD, and in the United Kingdom a much larger study (the STAND trial) is currently being undertaken to look at whether a mouth spray formulation of medicinal cannabis currently licensed for multiple sclerosis (Sativex) may be helpful for BPSD. Clinical research is also being conducted in Australia – at the University of Notre Dame in Perth – again using a mouth spray. It is hoped that, with time, clinicians will be able to make more informed decisions about the use of cannabinoids in dementia.

Other medications

There are a number of alternative pharmacological approaches to BPSD. These include the use of analgesics, which can be helpful when pain is an issue. Opiates are especially powerful analgesics that may also have a tranquillising effect, which for some can reduce agitation. Unfortunately, they can have significant side effects, such as sedation, confusion, constipation and urinary retention. Other agents (including lamotrigine, topiramate and pregabalin) also show some promise, though the evidence base is not compelling at this stage. Melatonin may be helpful for sleep disturbance (see Chapter 17) and is well tolerated.

One finding with BPSD that is important to bear in mind is that their severity may spontaneously change, and not necessarily for the worse, with the evolution of the underlying condition. This means that anxiety, depression and agitation, for instance, may be present at one stage of the illness, and then diminish in severity as the dementia progresses. As well as being a silver lining, this is particularly relevant when discussing drug treatment, as it is always important to regularly review whether or not medications are required.

It should be noted that the above is a guide to the different medications commonly used to manage BPSD, and is not an exhaustive list. It is designed to facilitate discussions with the treating doctor to allow optimal, considered and safe practice.

The issue of restraint

One concern often raised by the loved ones of those experiencing dementia who reside in residential aged-care facilities is that *chemical restraint* is being used. This relates to the idea that an individual is being given medications purely for the purposes of sedation and to 'make them quiet'. This is an understandable concern, and there is rarely any justification for such an approach, although the behaviours that are being addressed may be rooted in psychological disturbance, such as anxiety. In such a case, are we chemically restraining the individual or trying to treat their anxiety? Sometimes this can be hard to clarify.

Physical restraint is another intervention that is sometimes used in settings where there is problematic behaviour. This may involve the use of lap or seat belts, bed rails or deep chairs with tray tables from which escape is very difficult. Again, there is limited justification for using physical restraint, and it is not without risk: immobilisation may lead to pressure areas, while attempts to escape may result in entrapment or strangulation, abrasions or bruising. For many, the experience of being trapped can also be deeply distressing and increase the likelihood of BPSD. Sometimes physical restraint is used to reduce the risk of falling, though in fact the evidence suggests that such measures actually *increase* the risk.

Restraint has complicated legal and ethical dimensions that are beyond the scope of this book. A helpful guide to this vexed issue has been produced by Dementia Australia – *The Use of Restraints and Psychotropic Medications in People with Dementia* – which can be accessed online. The recent Royal Commission into aged care has also recognised the inappropriate use of restraint as one of the most pressing issues.

17

Sleeping, Eating and Mobility

- Sleep disturbance is very common in dementia, and may include insomnia, oversleeping and reversal of the day/night pattern. It can be caused by the underlying disease or by other physical, psychological or medication-related factors.

- Behavioural interventions may improve sleep patterns. Medications should be used cautiously due to potential side effects such as sedation and increased risk of falls.

- Dementia can cause numerous eating-related changes, including undereating and overeating, a narrowing of dietary preferences, and the ingestion of inappropriate substances.

- Medications, physical health problems and psychological problems can contribute to disordered eating.

- Mobility declines both with age and with dementia, especially in the later stages.

- Pain, sensory deficits (especially visual), balance difficulties and visuospatial deficits can all contribute to poor mobility.

- Mobility aids such as wheelie walkers may promote safe mobilisation. Physiotherapists and occupational therapists can provide useful advice.

Sleeping, eating and moving are among the most basic of human functions, and yet are not immune to disturbance in those with dementia. Sleep, in particular, is something I am often asked to help with – especially poor overnight sleep, which may be associated with nocturnal wandering and daytime lethargy. Dietary changes are also common, and the risk of falls is ever-present. This chapter describes the spectrum of changes and what can be done about them.

Sleep disturbance

Individuals with dementia commonly present with sleep difficulties. These include sleeping too much at night (*hypersomnia*), trouble getting off to sleep (*sleep onset* or *initial insomnia*), difficulties staying asleep (*sleep maintenance* or *middle insomnia*), reversal of the usual day/ night pattern (*circadian rhythm disturbance*) and daytime somnolence. This can have an impact not only on the individual with the problem, but also on the carer, who may be worn down by the need to attend to a loved one who is up night after night.

Causes

The underlying disease process causing dementia can directly cause sleep problems by degrading the circuitry underpinning the control of sleep and our circadian rhythms, as well as by reducing the amount of *melatonin* that is released. Melatonin is a hormone produced by the pineal gland in the brain in response to environmental changes – chiefly, when it becomes darker. It prepares our bodies for sleep. Natural melatonin production decreases as we age, and this reduced production is amplified in dementia. The message for us to go to sleep is therefore not as strong.

Sleep disturbance in dementia can also be an indication of other problems. These include the following, listed with some of their associated symptoms:

- *Sleep apnoea* – snoring, periods of not breathing overnight
- *Pain* – frequent awakenings, trouble getting off to sleep
- *Chronic lung disease* – breathlessness, frequent awakenings, coughing

- *Gastric reflux* – frequent awakenings, coughing, choking episodes overnight
- *Delirium* – fragmentation of the sleep–wake cycle
- *Depression* – trouble maintaining sleep, excessive sleepiness, other depressive features
- *Anxiety* – trouble getting off to sleep, agitation and restlessness during the day
- *Heart failure* – breathlessness on lying flat, needing to pass urine frequently overnight.

There are also a number of medications and other substances that may have an adverse effect on sleep:

- *Caffeine* can cause sleep onset difficulties
- *Alcohol* can cause fragmentation of sleep
- *Certain stimulating antidepressants* – such as SSRIs and venlafaxine – may reduce total sleep time
- *Lithium* may induce daytime sleepiness
- *Blood pressure medications* such as beta blockers may cause insomnia, nightmares and daytime fatigue
- *Steroids* such as prednisolone and dexamethasone may increase night-time awakenings and sleep onset difficulties
- *Decongestants* can cause sleep onset difficulties
- *Antihistamines* may cause daytime sleepiness
- *Anti-reflux medications* may induce insomnia and somnolence
- *Painkillers* such as opioids may cause sedation and impair deep sleep
- *Anti-Parkinson's medications* can induce insomnia and daytime sleepiness
- *Antipsychotic medications* such as olanzapine and quetiapine can cause sedation.

Treating sleep problems

The approach to sleep problems involves addressing the underlying cause, as above, if one is identified. Other, more general measures may also be of help, as the following sections set out.

Sleep hygiene

There are general measures, commonly referred to as *sleep hygiene* measures, that may be of benefit for those with insomnia. These include:

- Limiting caffeine, alcohol and cigarettes, especially later in the day
- Increasing activity in the afternoon or early evening (but not just before going to bed)
- Increasing exposure to bright light or sunlight during the day
- Trying to avoid sleeping for more than 30 minutes during the day
- Maintaining a comfortable sleep environment with the right temperature (16–18 degrees Celsius), darkness and ventilation
- Avoiding heavy or large meals close to bedtime
- Limiting liquids in the evening (which reduces the need to pass urine overnight)
- Having a regular bedtime schedule
- Engaging in relaxing and not overstimulating activities before bed
- Rising at the same time each morning.

Medications

In practice, several medications are used to treat sleep disturbance. These include *hypnotics* such as benzodiazepines (especially temazepam) and so-called *z-drugs* (such as zolpidem), *melatonin*, *agomelatine* (an antidepressant that works on melatonin receptors), *sedating antidepressants* (mirtazapine and trazadone), and *sedative antipsychotics* (olanzapine and quetiapine). Also *Seremind*, which is a lavender oil preparation that is available over the counter in Australia, shows evidence of effectiveness in treating insomnia (and mild anxiety). It also has the advantage of being very well tolerated and not associated with sedation.

My experience is that such medications can be helpful, especially in the short term, though it is hard to predict who will be helped and how well tolerated the medication will be. Not infrequently they can cause grogginess the next morning (though this often settles with time), and sometimes they seem to have a paradoxical effect, increasing sleep disturbance or causing nightmares. Drowsiness overnight can also be a problem if the individual needs to get up – to go to the toilet, for instance – as the risk of falls may be heightened.

My usual approach is to try melatonin first (a dose of 2 milligrams initially, about one hour before bed) or possibly Seremind, unless there is compelling evidence of depression or high levels of anxiety, in which case I may use mirtazapine or agomelatine. I try to avoid antipsychotics for sleep disturbance unless psychotic features are present or there is a significant risk of aggression. I also try to avoid hypnotic medications, as these can increase confusion and the risk of falls. Some individuals develop a tolerance, meaning that they need increasing doses, which also increases the risk of side effects. If the sleep disturbance seems to be related to another psychiatric issue, such as depression or anxiety, then medications used to treat these problems may also help with sleep.

As with all medications, it is best to revisit the need for them regularly. Insomnia may settle after a time and medications may no longer need to be used.

REM sleep behaviour disorder (RBD)

REM sleep – also known as rapid eye movement sleep – is the stage of sleep during which we dream, and is a normal phenomenon. During this time our muscles usually have no tone, and so although we may be dreaming that we are moving, we lie in bed relatively still. In RBD this loss of tone is absent and we effectively 'act out' our dreams, resulting sometimes in violent thrashing movements of our limbs. As you can imagine, this poses a risk not just for the person moving but also for their bed-partner.

RBD is thankfully rare in Alzheimer's and vascular dementia, but it is common in other dementias associated with parkinsonism, including Parkinson's disease dementia and dementia with Lewy bodies; in fact, it may be an early sign of these occurring. This association seems to be stronger for men than women – one small study demonstrated that over 80 per cent of men with RBD eventually developed this category of dementia.

Sometimes, RBD can be caused by medications, including various classes of antidepressants and (rarely) cholinesterase inhibitors. Treatment involves ensuring that these potential causative drugs are stopped and that the sleep environment is safe (with no sharp or breakable objects nearby, for example). If medications are required, melatonin is best tried first; if this fails, low-dose clonazepam may be helpful. Beyond this, medications have limited evidence of their effectiveness.

Changes in appetite, dietary preference and weight loss

Ageing brings normal changes that influence what and when we eat; these are not specific to dementia, and can include a general reduction in the desire to eat, feeling less hungry and having earlier satiety (the feeling of fullness). These may in part be due to physiological changes such as a delay in gastric emptying (how long it takes for food to leave the stomach) or changes in the part of the nervous system that regulates metabolic processes.

Our sense of taste also appears to deteriorate the older we are, meaning that we gain less pleasure from food. In addition, being less active means we do not 'work up an appetite' as readily as when we were younger. Older people are also more likely to be on medications that reduce appetite, or to have medical problems that result in the same problem. Poor dentition, including ill-fitting dentures, may also influence what we want to eat.

In dementia, these same factors influence the desire to eat and may be more pronounced. Exacerbating this problem, however, may be the loss of awareness of usual routine (forgetting that you should be having lunch, for instance), increased sensory deficits (especially taste and smell), increased distractibility or anxiety (meaning that you are less likely to sit down to finish a meal) and the inability to shop or prepare food. Many patients of mine who live alone have experienced marked weight loss in the months before I see them for the first time for these reasons.

Depression can also reduce appetite and occurs more commonly in dementia. There may also be specific problems with swallowing or chewing – particularly later in the course of the disease.

Disturbances in eating patterns in dementia either relate to loss of appetite/desire to eat, overeating, an uncharacteristic preference for eating sweet foods, or the eating of inappropriate and/or inedible substances.

Frontotemporal dementia seems to be particularly associated with disordered eating, with perhaps 60 per cent of individuals with this condition presenting with some kind of eating problem. Although there may be a number of reasons for this finding, it may relate to poor executive function. Specific symptoms include increased rigidity about what foods are eaten (potentially leading to poor nutrition) and globally increased oral intake (hyperphagia) – perhaps related to poor impulse control, and potentially resulting in significant weight gain. A preference for sweet and sugary foods is also a common finding and can cause metabolic and weight concerns.

The approach to eating disorders depends on the nature of the problem. Undereating should be discussed with the treating doctor to ensure there's no physical (including dental) or psychological health problem, and that medications are not causing the problem. Increasing exercise may stimulate the appetite, and being flexible about eating times may help. Offering foods that the individual is known to enjoy may at least ensure adequate calories. Creating a relaxed eating environment can also help. If there is prolonged undereating, there may be a need to consult the doctor about vitamin supplementation. Ensuring that dentition is healthy and that dentures fit well is also important. Having 'finger foods' readily available in the environment may help ensure that those who are too restless to eat a whole meal at least obtain some calories. In some cases, nutrient drinks (such as Ensure) can support weight and adequate nutrition.

Overeating may be helped by restricting access to food supplies, especially unhealthy snacks. Using distraction – such as going for a walk or engaging in another activity – can also help. Providing small meals more frequently over the day may be beneficial. Again, it is important to consider the possibility that medications are causing the increased appetite – particularly steroids, some antipsychotics (olanzapine and quetiapine) and some antidepressants (mirtazapine) – and this should be discussed with the treating doctor.

Dieticians are often very helpful when there are problems with undereating or overeating. They may advise the use of supplement drinks if there is substantial weight loss.

Eating of substances of no nutritional value may also occur. This is known as *pica* and can be both distressing to onlookers as well as potentially harmful – some substances can be toxic to the body, or potentially pose a choking hazard. I have known some patients with this unfortunate condition to eat hair, dirt, pieces of wood and even their own faeces (known as *coprophagia*). There is limited evidence about drug treatments in pica, though haloperidol, an older-style antipsychotic, has been shown to be helpful for coprophagia. Gentle distraction and limiting access to harmful objects is likely to be the most helpful intervention.

Mobility

There is a natural decline in mobility – our capacity to move and walk – as we age, and this seems to be exacerbated in dementia. The rate of decline appears to accelerate as the underlying dementia worsens. There is also some evidence that non-Alzheimer's dementia, especially vascular dementia, is associated with a faster rate of decline in mobility than in Alzheimer's disease. Certainly, problems with mobility are not a common accompaniment of early Alzheimer's disease, and if this is one of the first symptoms, other causes should be considered. Subcortical dementias such as Parkinson's disease, Huntington's disease and dementia with Lewy bodies are often associated with early changes in walking (gait), as is hydrocephalus.

Several factors may contribute to the deterioration in mobility associated with dementia, increasing the risk of falls. These include:

- A loss of balance and awareness of where various body parts are in space (proprioception)
- A loss of muscle tone
- Impairment of senses, especially vision, and difficulty processing visual stimuli
- The use of medications for other physical or psychological illnesses, which may cause sedation, dizziness or low blood

pressure, especially when standing up (these include medications used for high blood pressure as well as antipsychotics)

- Pain.

Concerns regarding mobility may be exacerbated by certain psychological and behavioural symptoms that may accompany dementia, most notably anxiety, agitation and restlessness.

In addition to the risk of falls – with the attendant risk of fractures, head injuries and other serious injuries – impaired mobility can lead to the individual staying in one place for prolonged periods, which can lead to the development of pressure areas or pressure sores. If these are not adequately addressed, they can develop into painful ulcers. Prolonged immobility can also cause other problems, such as blood clots in the leg (which can then travel to the heart or lungs) and chest infections.

Once reversible causes of poor mobility have been excluded, management of the problem involves maintaining lower-limb muscle mass by moving regularly. Going for daily walks can be beneficial, as can engaging in resistance work – such as with weights at the gym. If there are concerns about the safety of an exercise routine (because of cardiac or respiratory disease, for instance), an exercise physiologist can be consulted. A physiotherapist can also be very helpful, providing specific tailored exercises and advice about how to approach this. A walking aid such as a walking stick or four-wheeled walker may be required. Sometimes, soft protective helmets are used to safeguard against serious head injury, and hip protectors may be worn to reduce the risk of hip fracture.

It may also be feasible to make modifications to the physical environment to help reduce the risk of falls. This might include installing hand rails or aids to help a person get into and out of the bath or shower. Advice about such modifications may be sought from an occupational therapist, who can visit the home and look at the specific concerns.

In Australia, physiotherapists and occupational therapists can be accessed privately, though their services are also subsidised by Medicare – all you need is a referral from your GP.

18

Continence, Urinary Tract Infections and Sexuality

- Loss of bowel and bladder control is common in the later stages of dementia.

- Environmental factors can contribute to the problem of incontinence, as can physical health issues and medications.

- Toileting schedules and other practical strategies can help with incontinence.

- Urinary tract infections are common in those with dementia, especially women, and cause an increase in BPSD and confusion.

- Dementia can affect sexual behaviour in a number of ways: people may experience a loss of sex drive, increased sex drive and/or sexual disinhibition.

- What may seem sexual in nature may be about another unmet need.

- If there is any concern about sexual coercion or aggression, tell someone.

In this chapter, we will discuss changes in bowel and bladder function that may arise with dementia, as well as the vexed issue of sexuality.

Continence

Continence is the ability to control our bladder or bowel, and the loss of this control – otherwise known as *urinary* or *faecal incontinence*, respectively – is a common accompaniment of dementia, especially in the later stages, though it can also result from a number of other age-related conditions, including cancer, diabetes, heart disease, gynaecological changes, prostate enlargement, obesity and constipation (which can lead to *overflow diarrhoea*, when liquid faeces pass around the hard stool). It can be distressing not only for the person experiencing it but also for their carer and is not infrequently the reason someone has to enter care.

In order to maintain continence, an individual must possess the 'four Ms': *mobility*, *manual dexterity*, *mental capacity* and *motivation*. All of these can be compromised in dementia.

Contributing factors to an individual with dementia experiencing incontinence may include:

- Not recognising the need to go to the toilet
- Not being able to communicate the need to go to the toilet
- Difficulty undressing on time due to poor cognition and praxis
- Forgetting what to do when they get to the toilet
- Not knowing where the toilet is
- Being more susceptible to urinary tract infections due to prostate or gynaecological changes, or poor hygiene
- Being more prone to the effects of medications which may cause a change in bowel habit (constipation or diarrhoea)
- Impaired mobility.

A number of prescribed medications may also contribute to incontinence, and it can be helpful to determine whether there is a temporal link between starting these medications and the onset of the incontinence. Such medications include:

- Certain blood-pressure medications called alpha-blockers (such as prazosin and clonidine)

- Other blood-pressure medications called calcium-channel blockers and ACE-inhibitors (such as amlodipine, diltiazem, verapamil, felodipine, nifedipine, ramipril and enalapril)
- Some older-style antipsychotics (such as haloperidol, chlorpromazine, thioridazine, trifluoperazine and pimozide)
- Some antidepressants (through urinary retention – inability of the urine to exit the bladder fully – causing overflow urinary incontinence)
- Diuretics (these are often used for heart failure or swelling of the legs, known as oedema; their mechanism of action is to increase the formation of urine in the kidneys, and it is therefore not surprising that this may cause incontinence)
- Any medication that has a sedative effect, as these may impair mobility and increase incontinence; benzodiazepines in particular (such as diazepam, oxazepam and lorazepam) are problematic as they also relax the bladder, and this can then lead to involuntary loss of urine.

Of course, these medications may need to be used, and it is important to discuss the decision with your treating doctor before coming off any of them.

Treatment of urinary tract infections is an important part of managing urinary incontinence and is discussed below.

The National Institute of Nursing Research provides some useful advice on managing incontinence, detailing a number of different approaches:

- *Prompted toileting.* This involves encouraging the individual to use the toilet on a regular schedule, and providing positive reinforcement when they do. This intervention is more effective when they have an awareness of the need to go to the toilet. In practice, approaching the person every two hours and asking whether they are wet or soiled can be helpful as this draws their attention to their bladder or bowel. They then need to be checked and praise given (in a matter-of-fact manner) if there have been no accidents. The person is then asked if they need to use the toilet; if the response is yes, they should be helped; if they say no, there should be gentle encouragement for them to go anyway.

- *Scheduled toileting.* This involves taking the person to the toilet on a fixed schedule. Again, every two hours is a reasonable frequency, though this can be adjusted depending on observations about how often the person is passing urine or emptying their bowels. Trips to the toilet should occur first thing in the morning, at regular intervals throughout the day, before any daytime nap and again before bedtime. If the problem is faecal incontinence rather than urinary incontinence, the frequency of trips to the toilet can be less.

- *Habit training.* This involves observing an individual's habits in relation to how often they go to the toilet. In tandem with these observations, checks should be made as to whether the person is wet or dry at the time they usually would go. A schedule can then be developed, with the idea that the person is encouraged or taken to the toilet ten minutes before their usual time of need.

- *Fluid adjustment.* In general, individuals with dementia drink less than those without, and it is important to ensure they drink enough (generally six to eight glasses of water per day). If they drink more than this, however, it may be helpful from a continence perspective to reduce the intake. Providing the fluid during the day rather than in the evening or before bed may help with overnight incontinence. Caffeine (found in coffee, tea and many soft drinks) may function as a diuretic (that is, it increases the need to urinate), and so limiting its intake may be of benefit.

- *Dietary adjustments.* This is most relevant for faecal incontinence and involves ensuring that the individual has enough fibre (roughage) in their diet. It is recommended that individuals eat 25 grams of fibre per day; this can sometimes be hard to achieve through diet alone. Certain supplements (such as psyllium, sold under the brand name Metamucil) can help ensure adequate fibre intake. Observing the response to foods may also help determine whether certain foods are more likely to induce constipation or diarrhoea, though this is an area not well studied.

- *Rectal emptying.* This may help with faecal incontinence that occurs as a consequence of constipation. Hard stool in the rectum can stretch the muscles that usually prevent faecal leakage. This stretching weakens the muscles and over time they cannot do their job. Rectal emptying can be facilitated by gentle lower-abdominal massage, using certain softening foods (such as prunes) or consuming more fibre.

It is important that the toileting environment is as stress-free as possible, to maximise the chances of the person going at the intended time. Having the toilet room clearly marked can be helpful, as can making the toilet itself obvious – for instance, by having the seat a distinctive colour. Being vigilant to the signs of needing to go (sometimes just restlessness, or, in women, pulling up their skirt) is important. The toilet room should be well lit, including at night. Mirrors can sometimes cause confusion and distress as the individual may not recognise themselves. Having the ability to cover them may help.

Other general measures that may be helpful include the use of simple clothing (with zips or Velcro fasteners rather than buttons) to allow easy undressing, and ensuring that the path to the toilet is well lit, obvious and uncluttered.

Although there are medications that can be useful for urinary incontinence (by increasing the muscle tone in the bladder; one example is oxybutynin), these can worsen cognition in dementia and I avoid them if possible.

Medications for faecal incontinence are better tolerated, and can be helpful when the problem is related to constipation with overflow. These medications include stool softeners (such as docusate and lactulose), medications that add fibre (such as Metamucil and Benefiber), stimulants (including Dulcolax and Senna – these should be reserved for more severe cases), suppositories (for instance, glycerol capsules inserted into the anus) and enemas (for constipation that is more difficult to treat). Use of these agents should be discussed with the treating doctor.

Although it needs to be handled sensitively, the use of *incontinence aids* (absorbent pads or nappies) can be very helpful – especially overnight, along with the use of absorbent pads on the bed. You may be able to get help covering the costs of such items. Phoning the National Continence Helpline (see the Appendix for further details) will clarify this. Nocturnal incontinence can also be minimised by reducing fluids, caffeine products and alcohol close to bedtime. For men, having a commode or bedside urinal may be helpful. Keeping a night-light on in the toilet room can be of help too.

Urinary tract infections (UTIs)

In my experience, one of the most common health problems that individuals with dementia – particularly women – suffer are infections of the urinary tract. These can be problematic both in terms of the direct symptoms – exacerbation of incontinence, pain or discomfort on urinating, frequency of urination – and because they can exacerbate BPSD and cause delirium. They may also cause an individual to become seriously medically unwell, especially if the infection spreads to the kidneys or into the blood (*sepsis*).

UTIs can be recognised by offensive-smelling urine or changes in toileting. Sometimes an infection may be silent – that is, not causing specific urinary symptoms – but suspected because of behavioural changes or increased confusion. UTIs are generally easy to confirm with a urine sample (assuming this can be obtained), and they respond well to antibiotics. Measures to reduce the risk of UTIs include ensuring that the individual at risk is drinking enough fluids and that their personal hygiene is adequately addressed (including wiping from front to back and changing incontinence pads regularly).

Not infrequently, UTIs are recurrent, happening on multiple occasions. In some cases low-dose preventative antibiotics may help reduce the frequency of attacks. Cranberry juice is also sometimes used, though the evidence for its effectiveness is mixed and it can be quite unpalatable.

Sexuality

Sexuality does not vanish with age: it has been estimated that between 50 and 80 per cent of couples over the age of 60 are sexually active at least once a month, and that sexual activity continues throughout the seventh and eighth decades. It is also part of human nature to desire and seek connection with others. This may occur in a number of ways, from simple conversations and sharing of personal thoughts and feelings, to more physical acts that occur along a spectrum of intimacy: from holding hands, hugging and kissing to more overtly sexual acts such as fondling and intercourse. Our sexuality is an integral part of our nature, and can be expressed in many ways, including the way we dress, our manner of interacting with others, masturbation and intercourse.

It is wrong to suppose that dementia automatically removes the above needs, but their manifestations may differ – and in some cases may be a cause for concern. Because there are numerous dimensions to sexuality – physical, emotional and moral – it can be a difficult situation to discuss, but it is important to be able to have a frank and open discussion about any issues that arise. Emotional reactions may occur: anxiety, low mood, embarrassment and fear. The partner of someone with dementia may feel guilty about not meeting altered sexual needs.

Dementia can affect sexuality in a number of ways. These include:

- *Reduced sexual energy and interest.* Sexual drive is mediated by the hormone testosterone, the production of which declines as we age; it appears to be particularly deficient in dementia. This can be complicated by the presence of depression, and by certain medications (especially antidepressants and antipsychotics) which may be used to treat BPSD.
- *Misrecognising another as one's partner.* This can lead to inappropriate sexual advances. It is not unusual for an individual in the later stages of dementia, especially when they enter care, to try to establish a new intimate relationship with the misrecognised person.

- *Sexually inappropriate behaviour.* Also known as *disinhibited behaviour,* this altered expression of sexuality may be embarrassing for family members, and can involve flirtatiousness with strangers, graphically talking about sex and taking off clothes in public. Shows of public masturbation can occur, which may be highly distressing to witnesses. These behaviours are often the result of loss of impulse control and social propriety. The behavioural variant of frontotemporal dementia, in particular, is associated with this problem.
- *Increased sex drive.* This can cause considerable friction among couples if there is a mismatch. Sometimes this may occur due to the individual with memory problems being unable to recall having had sex recently. Again, frontal-lobe pathology may be associated with this hyper-libidinous state.

Sexual disinhibition and hypersexuality can be problematic when the individual is at home with their spouse, but also in the setting of residential aged care. In the latter instance, if this is coupled with misrecognition of other residents as one's spouse, this can lead to problematic sexual advances to strangers (including co-residents). Often the recipient of the advances is cognitively impaired themselves, and unable to consent to being involved in such acts, which adds tricky ethical considerations and further complicates the matter.

It is important to understand whether a behaviour that appears to be sexual in nature is actually an expression of another unmet need. A person who disrobes in a public place, for example, may in fact be trying to indicate they need the toilet, or are too hot. An attempt to kiss someone, similarly, may indicate loneliness rather than being a sexually mediated behaviour.

Options
What can be done about sexuality-related concerns in dementia? Well, it depends on the nature of the problem.

Reduced sex drive is only a problem if it is distressing to the individual with dementia, or to their carer. If the concern is actually over loss of intimacy, there are a number of other ways in which this can potentially be achieved: by the continued use of (non-sexual) touch, for example, or by hugging or the sharing of experiences. It is important, however, that depression is ruled out as a contributing factor and that any medications that may be contributing to the problem are identified.

Increased sex drive is a problem if there is a mismatch between the sexual needs of the person with dementia and of their partner, or if it is associated with inappropriate sexual advances towards others. If it is occurring only within the context of a long-term relationship, then it may be sufficient, if the dementia is not advanced, to have a frank discussion about the concerns, and to consider ways in which the need for intimacy can otherwise be satisfied. If the person with dementia has limited insight into the issue, redirection and gentle discouragement may still work. Physical avoidance of the person during periods of increased sexual drive (which fluctuates naturally) may also help. Identifying medications that increase libido (such as some medications used in Parkinson's disease) is also important. People experiencing certain psychiatric illnesses, such as mania, can also present with hypersexuality, and this possibility needs to be ruled out. Avoidance of exposure to overstimulating media, such as television programs or films, can also help address the problem.

Sexually disinhibited behaviour, including public disrobing and masturbation, should be treated matter-of-factly and without judgement. It may help to gently guide the individual to a more private place, or to distract them. Having a practised response to others who may witness the behaviour – such as 'I'm sorry, my husband has dementia and doesn't know what he is doing' – can allay some anxiety. Angry or offended confrontation with the individual engaging in the behaviour is *not* recommended. A practical help may be to use specific types of clothing that open at the back or that do not have zips.

As noted above, sometimes these behaviours actually relate to other problems – clothing may be too hot, or cause discomfort or altered sensation in the groin area – and these possibilities need to be borne in mind. If you are a carer facing this problem, then sharing your concerns with someone you trust – although perhaps initially embarrassing – can help you in devising a management plan and making you feel less isolated.

The emotional toll

Regardless of the type of behaviour experienced, changes in the sexual relationship can generate feelings of rejection, anxiety, grief (at the loss of a normal sexual relationship), shame or guilt (for not being equally enthusiastic about sex). It is important to understand that it is the disease, not the person, that is causing the problem. Sometimes partners feel as if they are having sex with a stranger, which can be very discomforting. Such feelings are perfectly normal. The stress of caring for someone with dementia may also have a deleterious effect on one's sex drive and desire, and this also needs to be recognised.

At times, a person's increased sexual needs or disinhibited behaviours may be accompanied by physical coercion or aggression. Clearly, such a situation needs to be addressed: no one should ever feel threatened or coerced into doing something they do not want to do. If this is occurring, it is important that the partner urgently seeks the help of another – this may be their GP, another health professional, a friend or a family member.

Medications

Although medicalisation of the changes in sexual behaviour is a controversial topic, in my opinion there are times when such treatment is appropriate.

Certain medications (including benzodiazepines such as diazepam and oxazepam) can cause disinhibition, and such drugs should be avoided if those behaviours are occurring. Other medications, especially the dopaminergic medications used in Parkinson's disease, can increase sexual drive, and may need to be reduced in dose or even ceased.

Although there are no so-called 'gold standard' trials (double-blind placebo-controlled trials) on the use of medications for problematic sexual behaviours, a number of agents can be considered:

- SSRIs such as paroxetine and citalopram can work by reducing obsessionality and impulsivity, and may also have an antilibidinal effect, reducing sex drive.

- Antipsychotics have a theoretically helpful effect of blocking dopamine (the opposite of the Parkinson's medications). Quetiapine has been used successfully at low doses.
- Hormonal agents such as medroxyprogesterone acetate (MPA) and cyproterone acetate (CPA) can also be considered. These inhibit the production of testosterone. They can cause unwanted side effects, however, such as increased appetite and weight gain, fatigue, loss of body hair, hot and cold flushes, glucose intolerance, and depression. The hormone oestrogen has also been used with success.
- If there is evidence of mania, a mental disturbance that can cause increased sex drive, the use of mood stabilisers such as lithium, carbamazepine or sodium valproate may be effective.

19

Pain and Skin Integrity

- Pain is common in individuals with dementia due to associated physical problems, though their ability to communicate it may be impaired.

- Pain can sometimes be managed without medications, though there are a number of medication options if required. Some of these may cause side effects and this needs to be closely monitored.

- With age, our skin becomes thinner and more vulnerable to breakdown. The consequences of dementia may exacerbate this risk.

- Vigilance for potential damage to the skin is critical and there are a number of helpful strategies to reduce the risk.

Pain

As we age, pain is one of the primary determinants of our quality of life. Our odds of suffering pain increase as we get older and develop degenerative conditions such as arthritis. In addition, our risk of falling over or otherwise injuring ourselves also increases the older we get, and these injuries can result in significant pain in the short and longer term.

Pain is also under-recognised and undertreated in the elderly, in part because some assume that it's an inevitable aspect of ageing.

It is not surprising, then, that in those with dementia, who are usually aged and frail, pain is frequently present; perhaps up to 50 per cent regularly experience this symptom.

Causes

Dementia itself does not cause pain, but the medical problems often associated with it may. Complicating the situation, those with dementia, particularly those in the later stages of the disease, may be unable to communicate that they are feeling pain.

Pain can be the cause of many BPSD, including sleep disturbance, apathy, weight loss, depression, agitation and aggression. It can also increase confusion. It may cause resistiveness to care, and lead to immobility – something that increases the risk of other problems, such as chest infections and pressure areas.

Common causes of pain in those with dementia include arthritis, constipation, urinary tract infections, pressure areas from being in one position for prolonged periods, falls (resulting in soft-tissue injuries or fractures), dental problems and neuropathic pain (arising from the nerves and more likely to occur in those with diabetes, vascular disease or spinal conditions). Pain and discomfort can also result from immobility and simply not moving your body very often, leading to stiffness and discomfort.

Measuring pain

There are a number of scales available to quantify the degree of pain, which of course is a very subjective phenomenon. These range from very simple visual analogue scales (where individuals point to a picture that best represents their level of pain) to more involved self-reporting scales. Unfortunately, those in the later stages of dementia – who are most at risk – cannot comprehend the scales being used. In these instances, the assessment of pain is made on the basis of observations by carers.

One useful tool is the Abbey Pain Scale. This summates the observations of a number of different manifestations of pain, including:

- *Vocalisations* (whimpering or crying)
- *Facial expression* (grimacing, looking frightened)

- *Changes in body language* (fidgeting, rocking, guarding certain body parts)
- *Behavioural changes* (poor appetite, increased confusion)
- *Changes in physiology* (temperature, pulse, blood pressure)
- *Physical signs of potential pain* (contractures, skin tear, pressure areas and so on)

An alternative scale is known as the PAINAD Scale. (The acronym stands for *pain assessment in advanced dementia*.) This assesses similar parameters to the Abbey Pain Scale, though it adds breathing changes and how consolable the individual is.

Both the Abbey Pain Scale and the PAINAD Scale can be downloaded from the internet. A mobile app, PainChek, is an innovative solution to pain assessment and is well validated in studies. It takes a short video of the person and analyses their facial expressions for signs of pain. This data is used in combination with other inputted data to generate a pain score that can be helpful in tracking responses to interventions.

Treating pain
Treatment of pain depends on the cause. The approach to pain caused by constipation, for instance, is quite different to that caused by arthritis pain. Determining the cause is therefore an important goal.

Non-pharmacological treatment
A *stepped* approach to pain management (one that promotes the initial use of interventions that are likely to do least harm) is always recommended. Such an approach dictates that non–pharmacological measures must be tried first. There are a number that can be helpful in pain management.

- For arthritis and muscular problems, *massage* and the use of *heat or cold packs* may be helpful. (Heat packs, in particular, need to be supervised due to the risk of burns.) Stretching and regular gentle exercise may also be of benefit. Physiotherapists can help guide interventions in this regard.

- Sometimes simple *repositioning* (after a prolonged period of being in one position) may be adequate.
- *Distraction* from the pain and involving the individual in a pleasurable and engaging pursuit may go a long way to helping with pain.
- *Music therapy* has also been demonstrated to be effective. Although this might be undertaken in different ways, the basic idea is to provide a relaxing environment with soothing music that provides distraction and alternative sensory input.

Pharmacological interventions

If specific causes of pain have been addressed (such as relief of constipation, treatment of pressure sores, or antibiotics for urinary tract infections) and non–drug measures fail to provide adequate relief, consideration should be given to the use of short-term or long-term pain-relief medications (analgesics). Traditionally, these have been divided into three groups: paracetamol, NSAIDs (such as ibuprofen, naproxen, diclofenac and meloxicam) and opioid agents (such as codeine, tapentadol, oxycodone, pethidine, morphine, buprenorphine and fentanyl).

Note that the medications discussed here are referred to by their generic names. They often have multiple brands, which can easily be identified via an internet search.

Paracetamol

Unless there are significant problems with liver function, the use of paracetamol should be considered before other agents are used, especially if the pain is mild to moderate in nature. When used in prescribed doses, paracetamol is safe and free of side effects. It should also be noted that in someone with dementia and chronic pain, the regular use of paracetamol may be more appropriate than an 'as required' prescription owing to the difficulty of assessing pain at any particular point in time.

The decision whether to use other analgesic medications needs to consider more closely the pros and cons of their use, as many of them have problematic side effects.

NSAIDs

Non-steroidal anti-inflammatory drugs (NSAIDs) are helpful for moderate pain, particularly if there is an inflammatory component – for instance, pain that's arthritic or musculoskeletal in origin. They are generally more potent than paracetamol. These medications can, however, increase the risk of heart attack or stroke, and may cause gastrointestinal bleeding. They may also impair kidney function and affect liver function. These risks are related to the dose of the medication used, and the duration of prescription. They should be used with caution in those with cardiac, liver or kidney disease, and in those with a history of gastric ulcers, heartburn or bleeding from the bowel. Other common side effects of NSAIDs include gastritis, diarrhoea, elevated blood pressure and dizziness.

Opioids

Opioid medications are best reserved for moderate to severe pain; ideally they should be used only in the short term, and their need reviewed regularly. The exceptions are cancer-related pain and palliative care, where ongoing prescription may be appropriate. These types of medication are, in general, the strongest available, though the strength varies considerably according to which specific medication is used.

Opioids are generally given orally (by mouth, either as a tablet or liquid), subcutaneously (through the skin, via a patch) or intravenously (directly into the bloodstream, via a drip). Oral forms include morphine, codeine, dihydrocodeine, tapentadol, tramadol, oxycodone and hydromorphone. Fentanyl and buprenorphine are often given via a patch.

There are a number of conversion guides that provide advice about the equivalent doses of different opioids, but these are just that – guides. There can be significant differences in the way individuals metabolise and tolerate the different formulations. Of course, any decisions about changing the doses and types of opioids must be discussed with, and closely monitored by, a health professional.

Opioid medications are often very effective in the short term, though they can cause side effects that can be especially troublesome for someone with dementia. These include a worsening of memory and cognition, sedation (leading to an increased risk of falls), constipation, nausea, and vomiting. Impairment of breathing (respiratory depression) can also occur. This can be fatal, especially when the person is on other sedative medications. Opioids may also induce depression. In some, they actually increase the sensation of pain.

This style of medication can also be associated with dependence and tolerance. Dependence means that the body becomes used to a regular supply of the medication; when it does not receive it, there are unpleasant withdrawal effects (including agitation, anxiety, nausea, abdominal pain and vomiting). Tolerance means that with regular use, the body needs higher and higher doses to gain the same benefit. This, then, increases the probability of side effects.

Neuropathic pain

This is a specific pain that stems from damage to the part of the nervous system that modulates our senses and pain production. It is not uncommon in the elderly. It may be the result of brain-related events (such as a stroke) or peripheral events (such as damage to the spine or certain other nerves). Diabetes and vascular disease can cause this peripheral problem, as can spinal degeneration (by causing impingement of nerve roots as they leave the spine.) Cancer may also cause neuropathic pain, as may multiple sclerosis.

The pain associated with neuropathy is different to other types of chronic pain – it is often described as stabbing, tingling or burning. It can be intense and very distressing.

A diagnosis of neuropathic pain is based on questioning the individual about the nature of the pain – something that may be compromised if the individual has dementia. A patient's history (such as a history of diabetes or spinal disease) can indicate increased risk, however. Sometimes X-rays can be taken to assess bony damage to the spine, or an MRI may provide even more information about spinal problems.

Although paracetamol and NSAIDs can provide some relief in milder cases of neuropathic pain, other agents may be more appropriate. These include gabapentin, pregabalin and carbamazepine. Some older-style antidepressants (tricyclics) can be helpful, and there is evidence that a newer antidepressant called venlafaxine may be beneficial in high doses. All these can of course have side effects – often sedation – and there's often a fine line between helping and hindering.

Skin integrity

As we age, our skin becomes thinner, leading to potential problems. We are more easily bruised and our skin is more prone to being torn. This may happen with minor collisions with objects, falls, and even from just being moved when we are immobile. These tears can become infected and cause problematic and chronic skin wounds. Several physical health problems can add to this problem. These include diabetes and peripheral vascular disease, which results in poor blood supply to the skin and a reduced ability to heal.

In those with dementia, poor nutrition may exacerbate the problem, as may weight loss in general. Immobility can lead to the body being kept in the same position for prolonged periods, possibly resulting in pressure sores or pressure ulcers. These may be quite painful. Incontinence and soiling are also risk factors, especially if it is accompanied by poor toileting hygiene, including being kept in a wet or soiled bed for a long time.

Maintenance of skin integrity depends on a number of factors, including addressing the issues above. This may involve encouraging regular movement, or, in the later stages of dementia, frequent repositioning, or ensuring that the person is well hydrated and eating adequately. Pressure-relieving devices such as special types of foam or partially inflatable mattresses can be useful. Gentle emollients (lotions) can be helpful in keeping the skin moist and protecting against cracking. Dressings can be used when there is established skin breakdown.

Being vigilant for problems is key. This can include regularly checking the skin, especially high-risk areas such as those over bony prominences. Early signs of problems include patches of discoloured (red/pink/purple) skin, or skin that is warm, spongy or hard.

SECTION III
Caring and Support

20

Communication

- We all need to feel heard and listened to, even if our ability to communicate is impaired. Individuals with dementia may struggle with both verbal and non-verbal communication.

- How to best communicate with someone with dementia will likely have to change as the condition progresses. Our body language and how we say things are often as important as what we say.

- Sensory impairments are common in dementia. These hamper communication, and need to be corrected if possible.

- Visual cues can be helpful when language is particularly impaired.

It is a universal need of humans to be heard, to have our wishes known, and to feel that others understand what we are saying. It is, after all, communication that has got us to where we are in the world, individually and as a society. The converse of this is that when we are not heard, we often feel frustrated, angry, anxious, sad or even hopeless.

The process of communicating may involve speech, the written word, or various non-verbal behaviours and gestures. Dementia may have a profound effect on an individual's ability to communicate, robbing them of their usual effective speech or impairing their ability to use body language to convey meaning. It has been supposed that impairment of the ability to communicate may underpin many of the problematic behaviours and disordered emotions that so often accompany dementia. Individuals with dementia still, on the whole, have the desire to interact and communicate, even if they lack the skills to do so well.

Communication can be broken down into verbal and non-verbal elements. The words we use account for only a small percentage of communication in general (less than 10 per cent). Non-verbal behaviour such as our body language contributes up to 60 per cent, and the tone of voice we use accounts for the rest. Elements of non-verbal communication include facial expressions, eye contact, posture, appearance, gestures, personal space and bodily contact.

For effective communication to occur, those involved need to have the ability to understand what is being said or shown to them, and to respond in an intended manner that makes our thoughts clear. Problems with language expression in dementia may include being unable to find the right word, using the wrong word or having difficulties maintaining fluency of speech. Writing and non-verbal communication may also be impaired. There may be difficulty manipulating parts of the body, including facial muscles, to convey emotions and thoughts.

How best to communicate with someone experiencing dementia

To an extent, this depends on the nature and severity of the underlying cognitive problems. Clearly, in the early stages of the illness, communication may not be too dissimilar to communication with someone without the condition, the only difference being the need to repeat the communication in light of memory impairment, or perhaps to use less complex sentences. This is a very different scenario to communicating with someone in more severe stages, where little you say is likely to be understood, and where other modes of communication (such as touch) may be more important.

One of the important factors to take into consideration is that *sensory impairment* is common in those with dementia (as it is in many elderly people). It is critical to ensure that an individual is able to see and hear as much as possible.

Paralinguistic features of communication are those that relate to *how* we say things, rather than what we are saying. These are as important as what is being said, with the same words being said in different ways having the potential to convey very different meaning. It is helpful to be aware of these facets of communication, especially when we are with someone whose skills are impaired. Paralinguistic features include:

- Volume (loud or soft). Hearing can often be impaired in the elderly, including those with dementia. It may be necessary to use a louder voice, but not one that is too loud. If the person usually wears hearing aids, it is important to ensure these are being worn and are working.
- Intonation and pitch (range of frequencies in speech from high to low). Dementia can result in particular difficulty in processing high-pitched voices, and sometimes lowering the pitch may be all that is required to improve communication.
- Rate of speech (fast or slow).
- Conversational cues that facilitate conversation (such as 'mmm', 'I see', 'right' and 'hmm').

There are strategies that may be helpful in communicating with those with dementia, helpfully summarised by Fiona Sugden-Best, a UK-based speech and language therapist:

- Always approach the person from the front and make sure you are facing them when you speak to them. Do not stand so close that personal space is invaded, however.
- Give the person cues such as using their name or gently touching them before you start a conversation.
- Try to ensure the environment is quiet and distraction-free.
- Use short and simple sentences, with simple language.
- Speak to the person as an adult and do not speak as if they are not there.
- Allow adequate time for the person to respond.

- Try to avoid completing the person's thoughts or sentences with your own words.
- Repeat sentences using a steady voice.
- Encourage the person to write down a word they are trying to express, and to read it aloud.
- Use visual cues such as a pictogram that may have objects or activities drawn on it so that the person can point rather than remember the name for whatever it is they are trying to express.
- Use appropriate and sometimes even exaggerated facial expressions – subtle expressions may well be missed.
- Do not correct the person if they make mistakes.
- Encourage the individual to use any mode of communication that works for them, such as drawing or writing.
- Use touch to aid concentration, and be reassuring.

Patience is key to all interactions, as feeling rushed only impairs the capacity to communicate effectively. Maintaining a relaxed environment in which to communicate can also be of great help. Another important point to remember is that there is rarely any value in arguing, and that this usually worsens things. Instead, gentle redirection – to another topic or another activity – is likely to result in a better outcome. This is particularly the case when, as part of the dementia, a delusional belief is held (see Chapter 16). By definition, a false belief is not amenable to argument, and disagreement will probably only inflame the situation.

The timing of communication is also relevant. Confusion may be more pronounced later in the day, and conversations may therefore be better held in the morning. Fatigue, another aspect of dementia, may also mean that frequent but short conversations may be more appropriate than fewer longer ones.

Having an idea of what topic you want to talk about can also be helpful; being able to fill in what may otherwise be awkward periods of silence can reduce stress and facilitate communication. Carers, relatives and friends often struggle to know what to say to someone with significant memory loss. Memories from years ago are often better preserved than recent ones, so topics of reminiscence may be the most fulfilling. Many individuals may recall memories from their childhood and early life, and can gain pleasure from talking about these things. It does not matter if the conversations are recycled if they provide pleasure to the individual and foster connection between people.

21

Legal Issues and Advanced Care Planning

- Dementia can affect a number of skills that are critical for driving. Losing one's ability to drive can be a major psychological blow and can lead to increased isolation.

- It is important to have a conversation early in the dementia journey about driving and when it will be appropriate to stop.

- If the person with dementia has impaired insight into their driving ability, and the risks are significant, consider removing the car keys until the situation can be resolved.

- Drawing up a will and nominating a substitute decision-maker are legal processes. A solicitor can provide details about the specific requirements, as these vary in the different states and territories. It is important to attend to these matters before the capacity to understand them is lost.

- An advanced care directive informs others of your future care wishes and should be completed as soon as possible, even if dementia is not present.

- It is important to understand the requirements and nature of an advanced care directive. Discuss the matter with your GP – there may be aspects of care that you need more information about before signing.

As well as the cognitive, physical and psychological ramifications of dementia, there are also legal consequences. These largely relate to the issue of impaired insight and reduced capacity to make decisions. This can have an impact on various matters, most pertinently driving, finances, and decisions about health and accommodation. Clarifying legal issues is an important part of the process of *advanced care planning*. As the name suggests, this relates to making decisions about future care – what interventions we want in case of serious medical events, and who will make decisions for us when we are unable to do so for ourselves.

It is important to note that having dementia does not automatically render a person incapable of making decisions of a legal nature: many people in the early stages of the disease are perfectly capable of making a wide range of legal decisions. As the dementia progresses, however, there will almost certainly come a time when the ability to make sound and reasoned decisions about one's affairs is compromised.

In Australia, the general requirements for someone to be deemed legally capable of making a specific decision (that is, to *have capacity*) include that they *understand* the nature and effects of their decision, that they can *freely and voluntarily* make the decisions, and that they are able to *communicate* the decision in some way. With dementia, cognitive impairment can erode understanding, and language deficits may impair communication. Poor memory and executive function can also render a person vulnerable to *undue influence* – that is, they may be told something false by someone with a vested interest in a legal matter, and not be able to evaluate this adequately.

Capacity is *context-specific* – that is, an individual may be able to make decisions about some things but not others. Complex decisions require greater cognitive abilities than simple ones. Clearly, there is a hierarchy attached to the complexity of decision-making: an individual may be capable of deciding whether they want to have a certain simple medical intervention, for instance, but be unable to soundly decide about matters related to their will.

Capacity is also *time-specific* – meaning that it is only relevant to a decision that may be made at that time. In the context of dementia, however, it is assumed (unless there is an extra issue that is temporarily increasing confusion, such as a urinary tract infection or medication effect) that lost capacity will not be regained.

The most common legal issues facing those with dementia are driving, creation of a will and appointment of a substitute decision-maker.

Driving

Driving is one of the most dangerous activities in which humans participate, but one that many of us love and cherish. We need to use numerous cognitive skills if we are to remain safe while behind the wheel. These include:

- The ability to sustain concentration and focus
- The ability to react quickly to a changing scenario
- Intact visuospatial abilities (knowing where we are in space relative to others), memory and orientation
- Intact coordination
- The ability to inhibit impulses.

Dementia can affect all these skills. It can also be associated with a loss of insight, which is perhaps the most dangerous aspect of all: it is not uncommon for the person experiencing dementia to have only a limited awareness of their impaired driving skills, or to minimise the concerns of others who have witnessed their dangerous driving.

Having dementia does not necessarily mean that an individual cannot drive, however, and in Australia there is no requirement to automatically surrender one's licence when the condition has been confirmed. This may in part reflect how treasured this freedom is to most people. Losing one's right to drive can lead to a sense of isolation and loss of independence, and may have significant practical consequences. 'Popping to the shops' or visiting a relative can seem much more difficult when taxis or buses or other family members need to be involved. In addition to these practical implications, there are also significant psychological effects, the loss of independence chief among them. It is probably not a stretch to consider losing one's ability to drive a legitimate cause of grief.

For these reasons, discussions around cessation of driving can be difficult. Well-meaning family members or health professionals who recommend relinquishing this activity may be greeted with anger or incredulity. Such conversations can sometimes be helped if the following tips are followed:

- Have a discussion when all individuals are calm (not in the immediate aftermath of an accident, for instance) and ideally early in the journey of dementia.
- Emphasise that the impairment is related to the disease, and not a reflection on the person's previous driving ability.
- Acknowledge that relinquishing one's ability to drive can be hard.
- Comment that everyone will have to give up driving at some point.
- Emphasise the financial benefits of selling the car.
- Actively discuss alternative ways of getting around – for example, taxis (the individual may be eligible for a taxi subsidy to help with the cost), public transport, lifts from family and friends, and so on.

In my experience, many individuals are agreeable to giving up their licence. For those who are not, it is important that the matter is discussed with the individual's doctor, whether that be a GP or a specialist.

Clinical assessment of someone's driving ability is rarely straightforward. As doctors, we do not experience firsthand the driving skills of our patient, and have to make a judgement based on the opinions of both the patient and their carer, which, as noted above, may differ. Cognitive testing is certainly relevant, and the specific nature of the cognitive deficits needs to be considered, as some are more relevant than others; visuospatial impairment may be of particular concern, for instance, whereas language problems will not impact greatly. If there is any doubt, I often suggest a practical driving assessment (conducted by an occupational therapist), in which the individual is observed as they go through the process of driving. Even with all this information, however, the assessment of driving is not an exact science. A doctor's evaluation of risk may be subjective, even if based on past experience and research.

In Australia, once an individual has been informed they have dementia, they are legally required to inform their state driver licensing authority (DLA). (See the Appendix for contact details.) This is the case with any medical condition that is likely to affect driving, such as epilepsy or stroke. This usually triggers the licensing authority to ask for a report by the individual's doctor, and may mandate a practical driving test. If there is thought to be an immediate concern about driving, your GP or specialist should advise you to stop until a decision is made by the DLA. If there is not thought to be imminent risk, you may be allowed to continue to drive until this decision is made. If the DLA approves a licence after this process, it is conditional, being valid for 12 months – at which point a further evaluation is undertaken. It may also have certain geographical or other limits as conditions.

Creation of a will

A will is a legal document and needs to be established in consultation with a solicitor. The solicitor should be sure that the individual making it has the capacity to do so. If there is any doubt, they should ask for a medical assessment to ensure that the person has capacity. In practice, by the time dementia is usually determined, most individuals have a will in place. Legal issues only arise if the person wants to change their will or create a new one.

In order to be capable of creating or amending a will, one has to have *testamentary capacity*. The basic requirements of this are that the person in question:

- Knows what it means to be making a will
- Knows what assets (bank accounts, houses, shares and so on) they possess

- Knows who could make a claim on the estate, and what moral obligation is owed to these people
- Is free of any mental disorder influencing the disposal of the assets.

A person is assumed to have testamentary capacity (and indeed capacity more generally) unless proven otherwise, though there are various elements of dementia that can impair this capacity:

- Poor memory can lead to an inadequate understanding of what assets the individual owns.
- Paranoid thinking, which may arise in dementia, can also lead to decisions being made that would not have been made prior to the condition developing. For instance, if John suggests to his father, who has dementia, that he should consider moving into a nursing home as he is unsafe at home, his father may meet this with suspicion, even if it is well meant. He may believe John is just after his house and so write him out of his will. Such concerns are common among those with dementia and cause considerable anguish. The suspicion may be a neuropsychiatric feature of the condition (paranoia); again, will-related decisions based on these beliefs may be considered void.
- Executive problems may mean that the individual cannot adequately weigh up and process the various elements necessary to making a will, such as reconciling competing claims.

Sadly, individuals with dementia may be taken advantage of. Owing to their impaired ability to remember and weigh up the advice of others, they are more susceptible to pernicious influence. An example: if Fred wants more of his mother's assets, he may lie to his mother that his sister Mary has been saying unkind things about her, with the hope that she may write Mary out of the will. The mother lacks the ability to rationalise whether or not this is true, and she may simply assume it to be the case. This would be seen as undue influence and may render her wishes as expressed in the will legally void.

Once a will has been made, it is important that someone other than the creator of the will has a copy, or knows where it is. Often the solicitor will hold a copy, though it is always wise to have another copy elsewhere.

Advanced care planning

There are two important elements of advanced care planning: creating a document that expresses our wishes about our future care, and appointing a substitute decision-maker. If they have not already been done, it is important to address these issues early in the course of dementia, as both processes require an individual to be capable of understanding them. Anyone over the age of 18 who is not considered incapable is able to do this.

Advanced care directive

This is a written record of your preferences for future care. It is legally binding. The nature and terminology of these directives varies from state to state. Here's an overview:

State or territory	Name of document	What it allows you to do
Australian Capital Territory	Health Direction Form	Write down your wishes about your future health care.
New South Wales	Advanced Care Directive	Write down your wishes about your future health care. Detail (but not appoint) a substitute decision-maker.
Northern Territory	Advanced Personal Plan	Write down your wishes about your future health care. Appoint a substitute decision-maker for health/personal and financial decisions.
Queensland	Advanced Health Directive	Write down your wishes about your future health care. Appoint a substitute decision-maker for health/personal decisions (not finances).

State or territory	Name of document	What it allows you to do
South Australia	Advanced Care Directive	Write down your wishes about your future health care.
		Appoint a substitute decision-maker for health/personal decisions (not finances).
Tasmania	Advanced Care Directive	Write down your wishes about your future health care.
		Detail (but not appoint) a substitute decision-maker.
Victoria	Advanced Care Directive	Write down your wishes about your future health care.
Western Australia	Advanced Health Directive	Write down your wishes about your future health care.

Many of these documents include not only your wishes about specific health decisions, but also about lifestyle preferences – such as where you would like to be when you are dying (at home or in hospital). They may include personal and religious information that is relevant to your health care and end-of-life decisions. As the above table shows, some directives allow you to nominate a substitute decision-maker, at least in regard to health and personal matters.

Unlike with a will, the creator of an advanced care directive often discusses their wishes with a trusted doctor (commonly their GP) beforehand. This can help clarify the ramifications of certain medical interventions that you may or may not choose to have. The directive needs to be witnessed, though the requirements of a witness vary between states: sometimes it must be a doctor, sometimes a legal professional, and sometimes someone else.

Specifically, an advanced care directive outlines what medical treatment or health care you would like to have if, in the future, you are unable to make decisions for yourself at the time. It can be general (for example, that you wish to receive all available treatments) or specific (that you wish to decline a certain medical treatment such as tube feeding). It provides guidance as to what you see as an acceptable quality of life, and when you feel it would be appropriate to cease life-sustaining measures – in the event of irreversible brain damage, for instance.

In a similar fashion to the other legal processes, an individual's capacity to create an advanced care directive hinges on their ability to understand the nature and consequences of their decisions (in this case related to health), to understand the nature and effect of the directive, to freely and voluntarily make their decisions, and to communicate them in some way, such as by speaking or writing.

A directive becomes especially valuable when there is otherwise some uncertainty or difference of opinion about what its creator would want. Different family members, all of whom may love the individual, can nevertheless hold very different views about the level of intervention to be applied in the event of various health problems such as a heart attack or stroke. These views may be influenced by moral or religious beliefs. There is often no right or wrong, but the differing views can cause significant tension among family members if it is left to them to make the decision. Often the decision also has to be made in circumstances where time is of the essence – it may be a medical emergency – and emotional distress can complicate the decision-making process. An advanced care directive sets out very clearly beforehand what the desires of the individual are so that the weight of these difficult decisions does not have to be borne by others. It is important to understand that the wishes set out in a directive take precedence over the views held by a substitute decision-maker.

There are a number of helpful websites and resources that give further information about advanced care directives; see the Appendix for details.

Substitute decision-maker

It is important for all of us to consider who will manage our affairs – be they financial, health or other lifestyle matters such as accommodation – if we are ever unable to do so ourselves. The person (or persons) we nominate becomes the *substitute decision-maker(s)*. This is particularly relevant where dementia is concerned, as it is likely that, sooner or later, the individual with the condition will need someone else to make decisions for them. As part of the planning process that comes with dementia, confirming the identity of the substitute decision-maker(s), in writing, is something that should be prioritised. Once done, this becomes a legally binding arrangement.

Although it may seem logical to have a single legal framework for the appointment of substitute decision-makers throughout the whole of Australia, unfortunately, just as with advanced care directives, this is not the case. The titles used to denote substitute decision-makers in the various states and territories include:

State	Name of appointee	Decisions able to be made by appointee
Australian Capital Territory	Enduring Power of Attorney	Finances and health
New South Wales	Enduring Guardian	Health
	Enduring Power of Attorney	Finances
Northern Territory	Decision Maker	Finances and health
Queensland	Enduring Power of Attorney	Finances and health
South Australia	Substitute Decision Maker	Health
	Enduring Power of Attorney	Finances
Tasmania	Enduring Guardian	Finances and health
Victoria	Medical Treatment Decision Maker	Health
	Enduring Power of Attorney	Finances
Western Australia	Enduring Guardian	Health
	Enduring Power of Attorney	Finances

You will note that the powers of a substitute decision-maker differ somewhat between states, emphasising the importance of discussing the details with your solicitor. Health decisions may include decisions about lifestyle more generally – for instance, where you will be living.

Regardless of your state or territory, there are important factors to consider when you decide to appoint a legal substitute decision-maker. Such a person needs to be over 18 years old, and they should be someone you trust, someone you feel will listen carefully to your preferences for future care and will be comfortable making decisions in difficult situations. You have to feel assured that they will make decisions based on *what you would want*. Individuals who might be appointed as substitute decision-makers include a spouse, adult children, siblings, friends and legal representatives.

The appointment of a substitute decision-maker requires the completion of a legal document that states who it is you want to appoint and the extent of their decision-making abilities. (Again, the Appendix provides more detail.) It is perfectly reasonable to have one person act as the substitute decision-maker for health decisions, and another, or others, for financial decisions. Often individuals may have more than one substitute decision-maker for certain types of decision, as this can share the decision-making burden. Similarly to a will, the paperwork when appointing a substitute decision-maker is completed in consultation with a solicitor.

It is important to note that the substitute decision-maker can only make decisions about your affairs *once you are deemed incapable of making these decisions*. Some individuals I have looked after worry that the appointed individual will take over their decisions as soon as they have signed the paperwork. This is not the case – the document only comes into effect when you lose capacity. An individual also has the right to change their substitute decision-maker by amending the document at any stage, as long as they are deemed capable at that time.

In order to be deemed competent to appoint a substitute decision-maker, an individual must be able to satisfy the following criteria:

- They can *understand* the information relevant to the decision of appointing the substitute decision-maker.
- They can *retain* that information to the extent necessary to make the decision.
- They can *use* that information as part of the process of making the decision.
- They can *communicate* their decision in some fashion.

What if no one is appointed?

In Australia, when there is no legal substitute decision-maker in place and an individual loses the capacity to make decisions, anyone wanting to become their substitute decision-maker needs to apply to their local civil and administrative tribunal. (Contact details for these tribunals in each state and territory are provided in the Appendix.) These tribunals are also involved in resolving disputes between individuals involved in the care of an individual lacking capacity. They have the power to appoint an independent entity to make decisions on that person's behalf – usually referred to as a *public guardian* or *public advocate*.

In regard to financial matters specifically, another independent body – the *public trustee* – may also become involved if no one has been legally appointed to manage an individual's affairs. They can become substitute decision-makers or provide advice on financial matters such as making wills and appointing other substitute decision-makers. Some states have slightly different names for their public trustees. A list of contact details is provided for each state in the Appendix.

22

Ethics, Consent and Elder Abuse

- Anyone involved in the care of someone with dementia should treat them in an ethical manner, ensuring dignity and respect at all times.

- Consent is the same as permission, and has legal and ethical connotations. It should be sought for any significant intervention, including the use of medications and surgery.

- Individuals with dementia commonly lose their capacity to consent. If this is the case, consent should be obtained from the person's substitute decision-maker.

- Elder abuse is not an uncommon phenomenon. It may take various forms. Some abuse is related to carer stress. The best response to abuse depends on the details.

- If you suspect elder abuse, there are a number of supports available to assist you in handling the matter.

Medical practitioners are bound by certain overarching ethical principles that guide our dealings with patients. These should apply to anyone who is in a position of power in relation to another. This is of great relevance for those working in dementia care, where the individual with the condition is in a position of diminished power compared with those caring for them.

Ethics

Let's look at the four basic ethical principles of all health care, and how they relate to dementia.

Autonomy

The idea behind autonomy, from the Greek for 'self-rule', is that we must respect an individual's right to make decisions in relation to their own life. In practice, this means that we should not interfere with the decisions of competent adults, and also that we must strive to empower those for whom we are responsible.

In the context of dementia, *competency* is the key issue, as the cognitive impairment seen as part of the condition means that this may be absent. Individuals with dementia should be assumed to be competent until proven otherwise, however. Also, although there may be some decisions that cannot be made competently, many others can be. As an example, an individual may be incapable of making financial decisions, but perfectly capable of deciding what food they want to eat.

Loss of autonomy is associated with considerable psychological distress for some, and is often equated with a loss of independence. Autonomy is a key factor of self-worth, and greatly influences an individual's quality of life. Feeling that we have some input into and control over decisions that directly affect our lives is an important aspect of dignity and our sense that we are respected as a person.

For all these reasons, respecting autonomy should be a guiding principle when caring for someone with dementia. It should also be noted that although an individual may not be able to make a competent decision by themselves about a certain issue, it is still important to try to involve them in the decision-making process – for instance, by including them in conversations about the topic, and allowing them to express their concerns. Additionally, involving people with whom the individual has had a loving and therapeutic relationship in this process may be a proxy measure to promote autonomy.

As dementia advances, competency is eroded to a greater and greater degree, and more decisions may need to be made for the individual. Sometimes this can cause distress for the substitute decision-maker, who may need to make decisions that will be upsetting for the individual experiencing dementia, but that are necessary to keep them safe – such as moving them out of their home and into residential care, against their will, if there is a high risk of malnutrition through self-neglect. In such a case, allowing complete autonomy may not be in the best interests of the individual. A tension thus develops, though this can be partly resolved by integrating two further ethical principles – *beneficence* and *non-maleficence* – into the decision-making process.

Beneficence
From the Latin for 'to make or do good', this ethical principle is probably self-evident in intent. Any interactions with an individual with dementia should focus on trying to create a good or positive outcome for them. We must negate our self-interest and ensure that the person with dementia is the principal figure whose interests are taken into account.

In the example of malnutrition above, autonomy would dictate that the person be allowed to remain in their own home if that is their wish – despite the risk of illness and even death – but the principle of beneficence suggests they need to enter supported care to be given adequate nutrition.

Non-maleficence
'Doing no harm' is another important ethical principle. Again, this can conflict with autonomy. If we know someone is at risk of falls if they remain in their own home, then allowing them to do so would be counter to the idea of non-maleficence, as we would knowingly be putting them at risk of harm.

Harm exists on a spectrum, though, and sometimes it is appropriate to *minimise* the potential for harm rather than eliminate it. A good example of this would be the decision to use certain medications to quell the aggression of someone with dementia to protect those around them. Such medications may cause harm to the individual taking them (by increasing the risk of falls, sedation or confusion, for instance) but the tailored use of the lowest dose possible, for the shortest period of time, with close monitoring of side effects, means we are still adhering to the principle of non-maleficence. Another way of resolving an ethical dilemma may be to try to do more good than harm.

Justice

This fourth principle relates to the ideal that we should treat all people equally, fairly and impartially. It will immediately be evident that this can conflict with some of the principles just discussed. If an individual experiencing dementia is aggressive, justice may demand action to prevent harm to others (the use of sedating medications, for example), though this action may not be beneficent or non-maleficent for the individual being treated.

Conflict between ethical principles can be partially addressed by establishing early on what the wishes of the individual with dementia may be in circumstances that may generate this tension. Of course, a requirement here is that the person with dementia is competent to make these decisions – highlighting the need for the situation to be discussed earlier rather than later. The wishes of the individual may be known formally, for example with an advanced health directive, or informally.

Situations about which an individual's wishes should be known may include:

- What are the things that would have to happen for you to be placed in residential care? This may include physical health problems, factors related to carer stress (see Chapter 23) or risk-related issues such as wandering from home or recurrent falls.
- What would you like done if you become aggressive to others? What personal risks are you prepared to live with (such as risk of falls and other medical complications of medications) in order to safeguard the safety of others?
- What level of intervention should be applied if you become physically unwell in certain ways? This should be covered in the advanced health directive.

These are only a few of the many issues that may need to be discussed, but the more an individual's wishes are known before they lose competency, the more the principle of autonomy will be respected – even if an autonomous wish may result in the individual suffering harm. When someone with advanced dementia becomes aggressive to others, their loved ones often tell me, 'If they knew what they were doing, they would be deeply upset,' and that they would prefer to live with the risk of over-sedation rather than physically hurt others. There are often no right or wrong answers, though future-focused discussions early in the journey of dementia can be helpful in reducing the distress associated with these ethical dilemmas.

In summary, despite the many limitations that we may face as carers, we can always apply an ethical framework to our approach, trying to promote as much independence and autonomy as possible, and treating the individual with dementia with dignity. The ideal is to promote good, but if this is not possible, then we should at least strive to avoid harm. At times these ideals will come into conflict, and there may be no ideal solution – and that is okay, as long as we are aware of what we are doing, and we try to implement ethical care as best we can.

Consent

The concept of consent is intimately related to the idea of capacity, discussed in Chapter 21, though it is important to recognise that consent has an ethical dimension as well as a legal one.

Consent is synonymous with permission. When an individual is providing consent for something, they are saying it is okay for it to occur. With the progression of dementia, consent issues become trickier, as the person may lose the ability to consent to things being done that affect them. *Informed consent* is a similar idea, though it makes explicit the requirement that the individual is making a decision after they have been informed of all the necessary details.

All the issues relevant to legal capacity are also relevant to consent. These include financial decisions, health decisions, accommodation decisions and decisions regarding medications.

It is important to recognise that consent is always required prior to any substantial intervention that may harm an individual (even if it is designed to help them). Medications and surgery are obvious examples. If the individual with dementia is unable to consent (and they should be considered able to do so until proven otherwise), then their substitute decision-maker (see Chapter 21) is responsible for providing it.

Elder abuse

Elder abuse is an understudied phenomenon, and we do not have accurate figures on how common it is. Much of the data comes from phone calls to abuse helplines, though this does not of course capture abuse that is never reported.

Abuse in this context can take a number of forms: physical, emotional, financial, social and sexual. Neglect is also a form of abuse. It is thought that psychological and financial abuse are the most common forms. *Intergenerational abuse* (that is, abuse of parents by their children) appears to be the most frequent type, and elderly women are more at risk than men. Spousal abuse (most commonly by a husband against his wife) is another type, and can sometimes be a continuation of a long-term pattern. We do not have strong data about the frequency of abuse in residential care, though this has recently come into focus in Australia through the Royal Commission into Aged Care Quality and Safety.

Factors that may increase the risk of abuse include high levels of carer stress (financial or emotional), carer drug or alcohol addiction problems or history of mental illness, a known history of family conflict, and isolation due to geographical, social or language factors.

It should be noted that elder abuse can also be categorised according to *intent*. Specifically, the abuser might be well-meaning but unable to cope, and the abuse a manifestation of their distress or anger. Or it may be deliberate, calculated and reflective of psychopathy or antisocial inclinations. Neither is acceptable of course, though the interventions for each may be different. Whereas the latter is likely to require removal of the perpetrator of the abuse, along with criminal proceedings as appropriate, the former may be better addressed by reducing carer stress, increasing supports and closely monitoring the situation. Physical and sexual abuse are criminal acts in Australia, while other types of abuse are assessed on their particular circumstances.

In some forms of abuse, there may be tell-tale signs. These include:

- Unexplained bruising, broken bones, abrasions or burns
- A sudden withdrawal from normal activities or change in behaviour
- Signs of fear and anxiety when around the perpetrator
- Sudden changes in financial situation
- Bruising around the genital or breast area
- Bedsores, poor hygiene and weight loss
- Belittling or threatening behaviour by the carer.

There may of course be other reasons for these signs, but it is good to be aware of the potential for abuse.

If you're in Australia and you have any suspicions about elder abuse occurring to someone you know, there is a national phone number (1800 353 374) you can call. Each state has its own support service for elder abuse, though this national number recognises where you are calling from and diverts you to the appropriate state service.

Asking about the carer's wellbeing can lead to an illuminating and helpful conversation about carer stress and coping strategies. Avoidance of blame, a non-judgemental attitude and being open to hearing what the carer has to say is generally advised if the abuse is not considered to be intentional. Confronting a carer without due consideration is not wise. It is best to keep notes as to your concerns, and to be aware that many elderly people do not want to 'cause trouble'. They may also be protective of their potentially abusive partner or children. Emotional support should be offered to the abused individual; if appropriate, they should be encouraged to contact a support organisation (see the Appendix for details).

A final but important point: if there is an imminent risk of harm, take no chances and call emergency services. The phone number in Australia is 000.

23

Minimising Carer Stress and Obtaining Support

- Carer stress is common, under-recognised and can greatly affect quality of life. Do not suffer in silence. Seek help from others – either family and friends or professional supports.

- Remember that the best way to preserve a relationship is often to spend some time apart.

- Phone My Aged Care to organise an assessment of your needs, as the government may be able to contribute to the cost of your supports. Do this early and recontact My Aged Care if your needs change.

- Be aware of what professional supports are available in your area. There are a number of care organisations that can provide monitoring, as well as hands-on and emotional help.

- Consider respite care; this can be a lifesaver.

When a person develops dementia, the focus of attention naturally falls on that individual and the needs they may have. Caring for someone with dementia (and indeed for anyone with chronic health problems) can have very significant psychological and physical health effects on the carer too, however. This phenomenon – known as *carer stress* or *carer burden* – is under-recognised, and yet it is one of the most important aspects of dementia care.

Informal carers such as family and friends should know that

there are a number of aspects of dementia that can make the stress of caring severe. These include the need to care for someone 24 hours a day, seven days a week, sometimes with no support from friends, family or health professionals. Sleep disturbance and nocturnal wandering may mean that carers get no respite even overnight. Then there are the physical needs: toileting the individual, helping them move, changing their clothes and showering them, even (in the later stages) feeding them. Complicating this, poor insight on the part of the individual with dementia can cause them to resist being cared for. This may occur on a spectrum, from passive resistiveness to verbal aggression and abuse or even physical aggression.

The behavioural and psychological symptoms of dementia (BPSD), as we have seen, contribute more to caregiver stress than the cognitive impairment itself or the increased physical needs. Delusions, hallucinations and depression are especially predictive of caregiver burden. A younger age of onset of dementia, as well as communication difficulties (dysphasia), also correlate strongly with increased carer stress.

Complicating the phenomenon of carer stress is the emotional dimension. In most cases, at least initially, the burden of caring falls upon a family member – either a spouse or an adult child. This person may see themselves as duty-bound to care for their loved one, and so may put up with a great deal before accepting extra support. They may believe that asking for help constitutes a failure on their part, or feel guilty that they cannot manage on their own.

Dementia can have a profound effect on the nature of the relationship between two people. Where once they may have been mutually supportive and capable, now one is dependent on the other, and is often unable to display the affection and gratitude that the other has been accustomed to. In later stages of the illness, there may be frank amnesia about who the carer is – a husband may not recognise his wife, or vice versa. The spouse may feel they are looking after a stranger – which can, of course, be highly distressing.

The carer may also develop considerable ambivalence towards they person they are caring for; they may even feel resentful towards them, and feel guilty about this. They may love the person but not want them around. Closely associated with this is the concept and experience of *ambiguous loss*. This develops when the person is physically present but not emotionally or mentally available. It can greatly complicate the grief process, which is a normal reaction to caring for someone with dementia.

A perceived stigma around dementia can also cause the carer to be reluctant to seek help from others. Making things even more difficult, the individual with dementia is often reluctant to accept professional supports, which is also understandable. Care provision requires intimate contact, and there is an inevitable invasion of privacy that can be difficult for some people to accept. Family members, sensing this resistance, often make the decision to forgo these extra supports, and instead try to manage things on their own.

Being a carer for someone often involves relinquishing one's own interests in order to focus on caring. The carer may feel they cannot leave the loved one, either due to the risk this entails, or because, as sometimes happens, the person with dementia becomes acutely distressed or anxious when they do leave. This then leads to increasing social isolation and further diminishment of the carer's own quality of life.

The impact of carer burden

Given all of the above, it is unsurprising that carer burden may cause a number of adverse outcomes for carers. These include:

- Increased rates of psychological distress, including depression and anxiety
- Increased suicidal thinking
- Increased feelings of anger, which may result in physical violence to the person with dementia
- Increased stress within the family unit
- Compromised immune function
- Increased heart disease
- Increased smoking and use of alcohol
- Poor sleep.

Chronic stress of any kind has negative physical and psychological effects, and carer burden is no different.

Factors influencing carer stress

It is important to note that other factors influence the stress of being a carer:

- Spouses may struggle more than other relatives, and female carers seem to suffer more than male carers.
- Older carers experience greater burden than younger carers, and those living in close proximity also suffer more.
- Predictably, those with less support have greater difficulty caring, as do those who have less experience of the disease.
- A poor relationship with the individual with dementia prior to its onset also correlates with a greater burden of care.
- A negative attitude on the part of the carer, and one that is associated with overt and expressed feelings of hostility and criticism, also predicts greater caregiver burden.

Looking after the carer

It is critical to know there are things that can help reduce carer stress. These include good professional and social support (from family and friends, as well as from care agencies) and increased knowledge about dementia, its effects and how to manage it. Knowing how to communicate effectively may be of great help (see Chapter 20), and good problem-solving skills can also be of benefit.

Education around dementia is a very powerful tool – it is one of the reasons I have written this book. A non-profit organisation called Alzheimer's Disease International oversees national organisations in more than 80 countries, and these can provide invaluable advice on dementia. They usually have websites that provide lots of information, and through these carers can discover local support groups and respite options. The Wicking Dementia Centre, part of the University of Tasmania, is also a great source of information, running free online courses. (See the Appendix for details.)

It is important that carers look after their own mental health. This means eating well, optimising their sleep (sleep hygiene measures can be helpful; see Chapter 17), having time to themselves, having interests in life other than their caring role, and scheduling regular enjoyable activities. Relaxation techniques such as mindfulness and meditation are very helpful for some. It is wise for carers to discuss management of their stress with their doctor, especially if it is severe. Sometimes medications or formal psychological therapy can be helpful. Dementia Australia runs a National Dementia Helpline (1800 100 500) that offers free professional and confidential counselling for those with dementia, as well as their carers and families.

What else can be done to alleviate carer stress?

Making an effort to address carer stress may not solve the problem altogether, but it can make a huge difference to the quality of life of the carer, and improve the relationship between the carer and the person experiencing dementia. As well as rallying family members and friends to the cause – people who can share the burden, either practically or emotionally – it pays to be aware of what professional supports are available. These may be as simple as employing a cleaner, or having meals delivered so that cooking is not an extra responsibility for someone already overwhelmed with caring duties.

There is a hierarchy of other interventions that can be applied as the dementia progresses. These can be divided into three broad categories: home help, respite care and permanent residential care. In the remainder of this chapter, we will discuss the first two of these interventions; we'll look at residential care separately in Chapter 24.

Help at home

Some families may be able to afford private in-home care, and there is really no limit to what can be provided as long as it can be paid for. There are numerous organisations available that can provide staff to help in various ways, whether this be to help clean the home, do the laundry, oversee medication administration, attend to showering and toileting needs, or simply to spend time with the person with dementia so as to allow the carer some time to themselves.

The cost of using such services – which may be required for long periods, and may increase in tandem with the progression of the dementia – can be prohibitive, however. For this reason, most carers seek help from the government to contribute to the cost of the care. In Australia, a government service known as My Aged Care aims to provide this support. To be eligible, the individual affected needs to be aged 65 or over, or 50 or over if Aboriginal or Torres Strait Islander. (See the Appendix for details.)

The My Aged Care website (www.myagedcare.gov.au) provides comprehensive information on the process. Essentially, it involves you, or someone on your behalf, making an initial phone call to My Aged Care, or completing a five-minute online application through their website. Once this is done, a preliminary assessment is made by My Aged Care about what level of support you may need.

Broadly, there are two possible support packages that are subsidised: the Commonwealth Home Support Programme (CHSP) and a Home Care Package.

- The Commonwealth Home Support Programme provides the most basic package, and may include help with meals, basic chores, showering and self-care, medication management and access to certain services such as podiatry and occupational therapy. It may also help with the costs of ensuring your home is safe and tailored to your needs, or provide domestic assistance. Community transport can be organised, as can opportunities to remain in touch with others.
- Funding for a Home Care Package is provided if you need more assistance than that given by the CHSP. The care funded is divided into levels 1 to 4, with a higher number denoting eligibility for a higher level of care. You will receive paperwork confirming what level of support you will be funded for. Home Care Packages can provide assistance with showering and self-care, medications and wound management, and may involve allied health services such as podiatrists, occupational

therapists and physiotherapists. Help with meal preparation may be included, as may help with feeding. Ensuring your home is safe and tailored to your needs is an important part of the package, and help may be available for walking aids. Transport may also be provided.

Depending on the outcome of the preliminary assessment, My Aged Care will organise for someone either from a Regional Assessment Service (RAS – for the CHSP) or an Aged Care Assessment Team (ACAT – for a Home Care Package) to come and see you, or the person needing care, face to face. This interview will identify your needs in more detail. Sometimes the initial phone or online assessment outcome doesn't adequately identify your level of need, and this may only be obvious when someone comes to see you. If someone from a RAS feels you need more than they can offer, they will organise for someone from an ACAT to visit you. In Victoria, ACAT is known as ACAS (Aged Care Assessment Service), though they do the same thing.

Once the level of care eligibility is known, the My Aged Care website allows you to search for support agencies in your local area, and to estimate the out-of-pocket expenses you will face. It is generally expected that you will contribute something to the cost of care, though the exact amount will vary depending on which care agency you decide to use. RAS and ACAT assessments do not generally lapse, but a reassessment can be undertaken if your needs substantially change.

Respite care

This term refers to the involvement of professional agencies to allow a carer to have some relief from their usual role. It may encompass only a few hours, a day, overnight or a longer period. Respite care can occur in the home (where someone stays with the person with dementia so that their usual carer can have time to themselves), or it may involve the person with dementia attending a day centre, an overnight respite cottage or an aged-care facility.

As with home help, respite care can be accessed privately, though this can be expensive. Most individuals apply for help from the government, and this is achieved in the same way as home help: by contacting My Aged Care.

Emergency respite care may also be appropriate, such as when a carer falls ill themselves, or when the person with dementia becomes suddenly unmanageable. The My Aged Care website can provide further information, and there are special phone numbers that can be called if this becomes necessary: 1800 052 222 (during business hours) or 1800 059 059 (outside business hours).

To access respite care, a RAS or ACAT assessment needs to be completed. If eligible, an individual can usually access up to 63 days of respite per financial year (and sometimes more, if the assessment reflects this). An ACAT assessment for respite care normally provides funding for either low care or high care, depending on what the needs are. As with home help funding, once funding has been approved it does not lapse.

Respite options are an important element of managing the care of someone with dementia, and of reducing carer burden. Although there can be feelings of guilt associated with using these services (as well as resistance by the individual being cared for), it can greatly help the relationship between husband and wife or between a parent and child, and prolong the period in which care at home remains tenable.

When I first diagnose someone with a form of dementia, I encourage them or their carer to have a My Aged Care assessment performed as a priority. There may be no immediate need for extra supports to be put in place, but circumstances can change quickly and unpredictably; the primary carer may become unwell, for instance. Having funding in place can mean that any necessary supports are available a lot more quickly than they otherwise would be.

24

Entering Residential Care

- Start a conversation early about when residential care might be necessary. Involve trusted others in the process to share the burden of decision.

- Although there may be a period of adjustment, most individuals settle into residential care well. There are things you can do to help this process.

- Do your homework before committing to a particular aged-care facility. Work out the costs and make a shortlist using the service finder on the My Aged Care website.

- Visit all the facilities on your shortlist and use checklist questions as a guide. Take someone with you to help you remember what to ask.

- Organise a meeting with a senior nurse and carer soon after admission to highlight any particular concerns, and to generate a specific management plan if one is needed.

- Learn to let go of the carer role, especially when it has been burdensome. You can still be a loving spouse or relative without being a carer.

The decision to enter permanent residential care, or to place a loved one in such a facility, is often a difficult and distressing one. It can generate feelings of guilt or failure on the part of the carer, and often the accompanying prospect of loss and separation – potentially from someone you have lived with for many decades. The aged-care sector can be complicated to navigate, which does not help the situation. It is perhaps not surprising, then, that often the decision to place someone is made only after some form of emergency – following a fall and fractured hip, for example, or hospitalisation for health problems related to self-neglect, or the breakdown or ill health of the usual carer.

Despite the inherent difficulties, moving into care can make a very positive difference to the quality of life both of the person moving and of their carer who is relieved of burdensome responsibilities. This chapter outlines how best to approach the important decision of entering residential care, in order to make the process as stress-free as possible.

Just like help at home, there are a number of private options for aged-care facilities in Australia, but these will incur substantial costs to the individual, and are beyond the financial means of most. The government therefore subsidises places in certain aged-care facilities if you are deemed eligible. These subsidies are paid directly to the aged-care home, and the home must meet certain criteria – so-called Aged Care Quality Standards – to attract these subsidies. In this way, you know a certain level of care is assured.

Eligibility for a government subsidy to pay for a permanent place in an aged-care facility is assessed through an ACAT assessment (see Chapter 23). This assessment only determines whether you are eligible for a subsidised place or not. The actual level of care you may need is determined by the aged-care facility when you visit them, using a tool known as an Aged Care Funding Instrument (ACFI). The outcome of the ACFI assessment determines how much funding the government will provide to the facility.

Anyone over 65 who is unable to live independently at home is eligible for a subsidised place in an aged-care facility. Those under 65 may also be eligible if they have a disability (including dementia), if they are unable to live independently and if their needs are not being met through other specialist services.

Most aged-care facilities offer different levels of care. *Low-level care* is most suitable for individuals who are mobile and need some care assistance, such as with personal care, laundry, shopping and cooking, and medication supervision. *High-level care* provides 24-hour care by qualified nurses as well as by personal carers; this is most appropriate for individuals in the later stages of dementia, and those with medical conditions that require a higher level of care.

Dementia-specific units are also available in many residential facilities. Not everyone with dementia will need to be in these specific units; they are generally reserved for individuals who cannot be safely managed in other areas of the facility. These dementia-specific areas are often locked to prevent wandering.

Many facilities now have an *ageing-in-place* arrangement in which all levels of care are provided under the one roof, meaning that the resident does not have to move facilities as their needs change.

What does it cost?

Once you have been sent the ACAT paperwork to confirm what level of care you are eligible for, the next step is to understand the costs involved. The My Aged Care website allows you to do this, and outlines what is taken into account when calculating the cost. This involves providing details of your existing financial situation, including whether you own your own home and what assets and debts you have.

The cost of living in residential care generally includes a basic daily fee that everyone needs to pay (usually 85 per cent of the old-age pension), as well as a means-tested fee that some will have to pay based on their financial situation at the time of applying. How much you have to contribute towards the cost of the accommodation itself is also based on your financial situation.

The My Aged Care website helps you determine whether you are likely to have to pay a means-tested fee or contribute to the cost of the accommodation by asking a few simple questions (such as whether you are a self-funded retiree or own your own home). If you do need to have a means assessment, the My Aged Care website links you to a form evaluated by another government department, Services Australia. This form (SA 486) asks more details about your financial situation and can be filled out online or by hand. Once Services Australia have looked at the form, they will send you a document – a pre-commencement letter – clarifying what contributions you will have to make. You need to take this to the aged-care facility you have an interest in to get a good idea about the overall costs of you moving there.

Once you have an idea about your financial situation, the next step is to identify which aged-care facility best suits your needs. Facilities vary in regard to the maximum daily living cost and the cost of the accommodation itself; the My Aged Care website allows you to compare different facilities in your area.

What to look for in a home

Although costs are important, there are several other factors involved in deciding which is the best aged-care facility for you or your loved one. The My Aged Care website provides some of these details – such as whether a home is low care, high care or both, whether it caters specifically for veterans, and whether it has specific services for people with dementia. There is nothing like visiting a facility to get a good idea of what it is like and how it operates, however, and whether it will be a good fit for you or your loved one.

When I discuss these decisions with patients, I generally recommend creating a shortlist, and then visiting a few homes before committing. It can be very helpful to have someone you trust accompany you on these visits, as they may think of questions that you do not. As mentioned earlier, these decisions often need to be made at a time of high emotional distress, which can affect our thinking about the matter. Having someone present who is a little more 'removed' from the emotion can be of great benefit.

It is helpful to have a checklist with you when you attend the facilities – this will serve as a memory aid, as well as allowing you to compare homes later. Such a checklist may include the following:

- What is the physical layout of the facility? Would it suit you or your loved one? Each of us has different tastes, of course, and facilities vary considerably.
- Are there places where you can sit privately and in peace?

- What do the staff seem like? It can be illuminating to see them 'in action' and observe how they interact with the existing residents. Do they seem patient, kind and friendly? Are they brusque, impatient or impersonal? This can make all the difference to one's quality of life.
- What is the staffing policy? Is there a registered nurse available at all times? How easily can they be reached? What is the ratio of nurses or personal carers to residents? What training have they had? The regular staff at aged-care facilities includes a mix of registered nurses (RNs), enrolled nurses (ENs), assistants in nursing (AINs) and personal care attendants (PCAs). Unfortunately, in Australia there is no current mandated ratio of staff to residents. Comparison between facilities may therefore be especially helpful.
- What can you bring with you? Are pets allowed?
- How easy is it to get a GP to visit you or your loved one at the facility?
- What sort of activities does the facility provide? Does it have outings?
- Are there additional services available on site, such as massage, physiotherapy or hairdressing?
- What happens if the resident's needs change/increase? Will they have to move elsewhere?
- How well does the facility cater for language or cultural needs? Are there regular staff who can speak your language? Are there other residents who share the same spiritual or cultural beliefs?
- Can you take the person out overnight or for a few days?
- How are medications administered?

The location of the home is also important, influencing how easy it is for family and friends to visit.

Some individuals choose to engage professionals in their search for the right aged-care facility. Known as *placement consultants* or *brokers*, they are in a good position to provide advice and can be very helpful.

A process of adjustment

Once you have chosen an aged-care facility, it is important to discuss the practical, emotional and behavioural aspects of moving. Again, having someone to share the burden with can be very helpful. For the carer or loved one, this process can elicit feelings of guilt, loss and grief. Similar feelings of loss and grief may arise for the person moving into the facility, and there is the added complication of adjusting to the new environment. This can be hard for anyone who has lived in their own home for a long time, though it is often exacerbated by cognitive impairment.

It is common for individuals with dementia not to understand what is happening to them or why they are being moved. They may think they are just there for a few hours or the day, or they may believe it is a hospital or day centre. This uncertainty can resolve fairly quickly or can last some time – perhaps even months. It may cause anxiety, depression or an increase in other BPSD. Staff at the facilities are generally aware of these possibilities and try to manage any difficulties that arise, though it can be quite confronting for the person who has placed them there.

There are several things that can help someone adjust to being in an aged-care facility:

- *Emphasising the positives* – and there are some – of entering residential care can be beneficial. These include the potential for increased socialisation and activities, as well as the relinquishment of the responsibilities of running a house and attending to domestic chores. Placement can also relieve carer burden, of course, and this can often lead to improvement in relationships. Individuals who may previously have been preoccupied with the care needs of the other can now focus on more important aspects of their relationship.
- *Personalising the room* can improve a person's acceptance of staying where they are. I have been surprised at how often residents' rooms are stark and clinical. Putting up pictures and photos on the walls and bringing in favourite bits of furniture may all help the process, and may provide a talking point for

staff and visitors. Having a music player with some of their favourite music is a good idea for some, and others may like to have their own TV. Sometimes a small fridge can be put in the room and filled with their preferred foods. It should be noted, however, that some facilities put a limit on what can be brought in; this should be clarified beforehand. Familiarity of objects is much more relevant than how new they are, and I generally recommend against buying new duvets, clothes and the like.

- *Spending time* in the company of your loved one with some of the other residents may facilitate the process of adjustment. If there is someone you think they might get on well with (ask the staff for guidance), see if a friendship can be nurtured. Having a sense of connection to the facility can make the situation a lot more enjoyable.

- *Talking with the staff* who will be looking after your loved one can be useful. The more information they have about the person entering residential care, the more helpful their interactions are likely to be. Have a meeting with the nurse and a carer soon after arrival to discuss things in your loved one's history that might make them feel more welcome. This might include recognising their likes and dislikes, activities they have enjoyed over the years, and their quirks and idiosyncrasies (which we all have!). Tell the staff what your loved one was like before the dementia to help the staff see the person *beyond* the dementia. A 'life story' scrapbook may also help staff learn about your loved one. This can be left in their room.

- *Identifying possible problematic behaviours* early on – BPSD that they may have experienced at home – and discussing these with the staff is important. Again, a meeting with the nurse and a carer may be helpful in this regard. It is often particularly effective to draw up a written management plan for these issues – one that all the staff can read and be aware of. Unfortunately, there is often a high turnover of staff in aged-care facilities, including agency staff who may not have met your loved one before. Having access to this written plan, which outlines the best approach to your loved one, can ensure there is *consistency* of approach. This can be of great help.

Letting go

Many spouses or relatives find it hard to relinquish the carer role once their loved one has moved to a residential care home. It is possible they have had this role for many years, and although it may have been burdensome and distressing, it often has become an ingrained habit.

Part of the difficulty of letting go may be driven by feelings of guilt about abandoning your loved one, or by concerns that the staff at the facility won't be as attentive or competent as you have been. Some spouses or children visit every day to feed, dress and shower their loved one. This is a vexed issue, and it is probably true that the devoted, one-to-one care that you have provided will not be able to be emulated in an aged-care facility, especially with the staffing levels that exist currently. It is important to realise, however, that staff have had training in the provision of care and the vast majority are well-intentioned.

It should also be recognised that often the reason that residential care has become necessary is because of carer stress. Unless you make some attempt to extricate yourself from this role, the burden may persist, and one of the advantages of placement will be lost.

Facilities and individuals vary in their response to what may be seen as over-involvement in the care process on the part of relatives. It is important to talk with a trusted member of staff about how involved you should be, and what the pros and cons may be. It is equally important to be able to respectfully raise any specific concerns you may have about the care that is being provided. Your own experience as a carer is invaluable, and any tips you have learnt that might help your loved one receive the best care should be welcomed by staff.

There is absolutely nothing wrong with wanting to provide some care – caring can provide invaluable opportunities for moments of comfort, tenderness and connection – but the balance has to be correct. Remember also that, in the end, most individuals do adapt well to their new environment and become settled.

Separating and saying goodbye

I am often asked by families how frequently they should visit their loved one when they first enter residential care. There is no single answer to this, as it is hard to predict a person's reaction. The obvious concern is that visiting too frequently will mean that the individual in care may become upset when the visit ends, or that the visits will be associated with pleading to go home – something that can be very distressing for the person visiting them. Conversely, the fear with not visiting enough is that it will make the individual in care feel abandoned and unloved.

The best approach is to try to find a happy medium between these two conflicting concerns, and usually that will only become evident after a provisional plan is put in place and the response gauged. Relatives are often surprised at how well their loved one adjusts to a change in circumstances. Being flexible, and accepting that the arrangement may need to change, is an important part of this process. Talking with staff at the facility can also help you make decisions about this.

If the person with dementia has been placed in residential care because of BPSD and carer stress, it is important for you as a carer to acknowledge this, and to allow yourself to have some 'time off'. This may mean that you visit less often than you would if this wasn't a concern.

Some individuals with dementia can find it distressing when their visitor leaves, believing either that they should be going with them, or that they are being abandoned. This can lead to increased agitation. Again, I am often asked for advice about how to handle this. Although there are numerous ways of managing the situation, distraction is often helpful. Letting staff know when you are likely to be leaving and asking that they occupy the person left behind with a task or activity can sometimes be helpful. Leaving at mealtimes often works well for this reason. I think it is important to always say goodbye, but in those who have very limited short-term memory, I also feel it is reasonable to be imprecise but reassuring.

25

Cultivating Happiness and Meaning in Dementia

- Dementia does not rob an individual of the capacity for joy or a meaningful life.
- Activities designed to promote happiness and meaning need to be tailored to the individual and may change as the dementia progresses.
- It is important to avoid activities that induce stress, and to remember that the goal is to instil positive emotions. The outcome of the activity is otherwise irrelevant.
- Even the simplest of touches and the briefest of positive interactions have the power to induce happiness.

In my line of work, it is all too easy to focus on the problems that occur in dementia, but something that has become increasingly apparent to me over the years is that the capacity for positive emotions – from gentle contentment to effusive happiness or even awe – is not inevitably lost with dementia. It is quite possible to have substantial impairment of memory or other cognitive problems and yet to feel happy.

From a neurological perspective, this is unsurprising. Although there is clearly a link between emotions, memory and other cognitive functions, the parts of the brain responsible for producing each differ. Emotions are often modulated by subcortical structures, including parts of the limbic system such as the hypothalamus, amygdala and limbic cortex. In the more common types of dementia, including that related to Alzheimer's disease, these subcortical structures are typically spared, at least early on.

There are, however, a number of challenges to happiness that may occur in tandem with developing dementia. These include:

- An awareness of deteriorating function and thinking
- Attendant physical health problems, especially pain
- Feelings of social isolation, compounded by poor hearing, vision and understanding
- Placement in an unfamiliar environment (such as an aged-care facility) due to increased care needs
- The potential for specific psychological problems arising due to the dementia – including depression, anxiety, paranoia and hallucinations
- Limited capacity for physical exercise
- Fatigue.

As we have seen throughout this book, knowing about these challenges can help us address them. It can also be helpful to remind ourselves of the main ingredients of happiness more broadly. These include:

- Feeling safe
- Having a sense of purpose and being actively engaged in meaningful tasks
- Having a sense of connectedness to others
- Feeling loved, supported and valued.

These are very basic needs, though profound in their implications. Dementia does not negate our requirement for them, nor does it rob us of the capacity to enjoy them.

How, though, do we achieve a sense of purpose if we or our loved one are experiencing substantial cognitive impairment? Well, it is important to remember that purpose does not have to mean something grandiose or world-changing – being occupied in the moment can be enough for someone with limited memory capacity to feel contented. It is important to know the types of activities that the individual experiencing dementia is likely to enjoy, and to avoid anything that may induce stress. With these caveats in mind, the options are limited only by our imagination.

Purpose means different things to different people. Examples of 'purposeful' activities will vary according to the extent of cognitive impairment. In my practice I have seen or heard of many, including:

- Gardening
- Journaling or writing one's life history
- Completing craft projects
- Helping with domestic duties, such as sweeping, folding clothes, sheets or napkins, washing up
- Being given some other 'helping' role
- Walking the dog or caring for pets
- Looking after grandchildren
- Volunteering.

It is important to avoid value judgements when considering activities. These are, after all, intended to promote happiness for the person with dementia, whose opinion may be (or may have been) different to ours. With impairment of memory, there can be much more value in a moment-to-moment experience than in any longer-term search for meaning.

Some activities may need modification – especially as the dementia progresses – but they can still provide great satisfaction, either in the moment or more enduringly. Individuals may need assistance when undertaking these activities, though this provides opportunities for quiet accompaniment by a loved one. This is often beneficial, as the focus can be taken off the need for constant conversation, something that can be a challenge. Being engaged in a pleasurable activity and surrounded by people we know and love can be greatly satisfying and calming.

Although it is a personal matter, there are a large number of activities and experiences that may be accessible and enjoyable for individuals experiencing the different stages of dementia. Here are some examples:

- Reminiscing on pleasant times and sharing memories
- Listening to familiar music
- Playing simple board games or card games
- Watching old family videos or going through old photographs
- Watching comedies (as dementia advances, more complex humour may be difficult to understand, but slapstick and simple visual gags may still be appreciated)
- Going for walks
- Reading magazines, the newspaper or coffee-table books
- Watching films that the individual has previously enjoyed
- Singing and/or dancing
- Visiting museums or art galleries
- Quizzes or wordplay exercises (especially in group settings)
- Enjoying a cup of coffee or tea with a loved one
- Spending time in nature
- Engaging in faith-based activities if this has been part of an individual's life prior to the dementia
- Massage, hugs or even gentle touch from loved ones.

When considering activities that might create joy or meaning, it is useful to understand the specific cognitive deficits that the person with dementia may have, and to cater to their strengths. In this way, there is less likely to be stress associated with the activity. It might be best not to ask someone with significant language difficulties to engage in activities where speech is a core component (such as a quiz). For this person, an activity that is more practical and hands-on (such as craft) might be more appropriate. Strengths-based activities are key. Sometimes it takes trial and error to understand what suits, so it is important to be flexible, both in the specifics of the activity and in the timing. Often, individuals with dementia function better in the morning. Activities informed by previous interests may provide particular enjoyment, though this is not always the case.

Having said all this, it is important to avoid asking individuals to engage in condescendingly simple activities. Likewise, the activity should be undertaken at their pace, not yours. A lack of interest indicates that the activity should be stopped, and there should be no emphasis on completing tasks accurately. If the person is struggling with an activity, gently support them with it, but do not laugh or rush or get anxious; if it causes any distress, move on to something else. Whether the task is finished or not is irrelevant.

Overall, it is important to recognise that neither the capacity for joy nor meaning are automatically eroded by dementia, and there are many things we can do to promote these crucially important aspects of living.

26

Dying and End-of-life Care

- Dementia is a terminal condition, and may itself cause death.

- End-of-life care is designed to allow an individual to live as comfortable and complete a life as possible. It may commence months to years before death is anticipated.

- It is far preferable to understand an individual's wishes in relation to end-of-life care before they are unable to make judgements. This can be enshrined in an advanced health directive.

- Acting as a substitute decision-maker can create understandable feelings of guilt or sadness, but being well informed, thoughtful and caring is the surest way to make the right decisions.

- End-of-life care may involve physical, psychological, cultural and spiritual elements.

As with so many aspects of dementia, end-of-life care has practical, emotional, legal and moral dimensions. This chapter seeks to discuss this important but sometimes divisive issue.

Coming to terms with the prospect of death

Dementia is a terminal condition, meaning that if no other health problem intervenes, the condition itself will cause death. Although this is not widely recognised, it should not be surprising when we consider the critical role of the brain in controlling our heart, lungs, gut and other metabolic processes. Although it is very hard to predict how long it will be before death arrives for any person, from the point of diagnosis those with mild dementia live, on average, between three and seven years, those with moderate dementia from 1.5 to 3 years, and those with severe dementia from 1.4 to 2.4 years.

Much like the common response to being informed about having dementia, the news that you or a loved one will die can evoke a wide range of emotions. These include shock or disbelief, sadness, numbness, anger, anxiety and fear. These are all normal. Feelings of loss of control may be especially harrowing, and concerns about the mechanism of death – will it be painful? How much suffering will there be? – feed into our anxiety about what lies ahead. What is important is that the person with dementia is both supported (by family, friends and professionals), and given time to themselves to come to terms with the inevitability. The experience is different for everyone.

End-of-life care

Also known as *palliative care*, this focuses more on the specific symptoms of a condition (such as pain or breathlessness) than on the underlying diagnosis. Cancer, heart and lung disease, stroke and dementia are all examples of conditions that may require this type of care.

Understandably, most individuals see end-of-life care as relating to the final hours to days to weeks of one's life, though it is best conceptualised as any form of care that involves a condition that is *incurable, progressive* and *at an advanced stage*. It may therefore be relevant for a number of years before death takes place. Implicit in this definition is the idea that end-of-life care aims to provide comfort to the person experiencing the terminal condition, and to improve quality of life for that individual and those around them. It is a support system to help an individual live their life as comfortably and fully as they can.

'Palliative care' is defined by the World Health Organization (WHO) as 'the active total care of patients whose disease is not responsive to curative treatment'. The WHO goes on to say that 'control of pain … and of psychological, social and spiritual problems, is paramount'. This highlights the multidimensional aspect of care, and emphasises that 'the goal of palliative care is the achievement of the best quality of life for patients and their families'.

One of the most important decisions around palliative care relates to whether quantity of life or quality of life is the most important outcome. Often the two may not be compatible, as some medications used in palliation, such as strong painkillers, can hasten death. It should be noted that this is not the intention of palliative care, which is designed neither to hasten death nor to shorten life, but that it may occur.

Other requirements are to establish what the goal of care is, and to make some determination about what to do in an emergency situation where an individual may require cardio-pulmonary resuscitation. These issues are important to discuss within the family, and also with a health professional – ideally a GP who knows you or your loved one well.

Palliative care may also be used to address medical conditions that occur independently of the dementia itself, such as cancer or chronic lung disease.

Who's involved in end-of-life care?

A number of professionals and institutions may be part of the team providing end-of-life care. These include GPs, medical specialists (such as palliative care physicians), nursing staff, allied health professionals, social workers, cultural and religious service providers, hospitals, aged-care facilities, and hospices.

Following the patient's wishes

Choices about palliative care, like all choices made in the context of dementia, are best defined (preferably in writing) early in the journey, when the individual with the condition is able to make sound decisions about the matter. These wishes can be documented as part of an advanced care directive (see Chapter 21). Without this, difficult decisions have to be made by the substitute decision-maker (again, see Chapter 21), often a family member who may be emotionally distressed by this challenge. The advanced care directive should be kept in a place that is known and accessible to others so that it can be referred to in an emergency.

If you are the substitute decision-maker, and the desires of the person you are deciding for are unknown, it will be helpful to put yourself in their shoes. What do you think they would want done? What goal would make sense to them? There are often no right or wrong answers, of course, and decisions are based as much on personal, psychological and cultural beliefs as they are on objective, factual evidence. It's important to recognise that the individual's choices may run counter to your own, but it is their opinion that is most relevant, not yours.

If the decision about end-of-life care falls to you, as a substitute decision-maker, you may feel considerable ambivalence. If you make a decision that focuses on the person's comfort, though one that also inadvertently hastens death, you may experience feelings of guilt or sadness. These are understandable emotions and do not indicate that you made the 'wrong' decision. As long as you can say you have acted in a thoughtful, compassionate and honest manner, keeping the views of the other person paramount, then you have done your job.

What symptoms might end-of-life care aim to address?

With its emphasis on comfort, it is not surprising that end-of-life care often involves assessing and treating pain. This topic is covered in Chapter 19. Opioid painkillers such as morphine may have a greater role in palliative care than in other instances.

There are a number of other symptoms that commonly need to be addressed during end-of-life care:

- *Breathlessness* (dyspnoea) is a subjective symptom and can be very distressing. It is common in late-stage dementia and can be related to general decline, respiratory or cardiac problems, infections, psychological distress or the side effects of medications. Reducing breathlessness may involve treating the underlying cause, the use of respiratory exercises, and repositioning the body and circulating air to the face (using a fan or fresh air, for example). Opioid medications may also be helpful in some cases.

- *Nutrition and hydration* are important aspects of end-of-life care, as reduced oral intake is a problem for many individuals with advanced dementia. The use of artificial feeding (with a nasogastric tube, for instance) does not have a significant impact on the survival rates of those with dementia and may cause undue harm (via infection, bleeding or gastrointestinal symptoms). Artificial hydration – for instance, via a drip – can be comforting, however, by relieving symptoms of a dry mouth. It needs to be done at a rate that does not cause fluid overload.

- *Mouth care* is another important aspect of palliative care, as poor oral hygiene can lead to problems such as pain, infection, ulcers and poor oral intake secondary to discomfort and difficulties swallowing. Oral hygiene can be assessed by a dentist or dental nurse.

- *Constipation* may also occur in the advanced stages of dementia, and can cause a number of health problems, including pain, delirium, urinary retention, overflow faecal incontinence and haemorrhoids. Medical emergencies such as bowel perforation or obstruction may also occur, and constipation may exacerbate BPSD. (See Chapter 18 for more information.)

- *Psychological symptoms* are relatively common and are understandable, especially when someone is aware of what is happening and that death may not be far off. They may respond to the regular supportive contact of others – both loved ones and trained counsellors – but may also be helped by medications that allay anxiety or improve mood.

A person's spiritual needs should also be considered as they reach the end of their life, though how to address this will vary greatly depending on their cognitive awareness. Spirituality does not need to be manifest as specific religious belief; it can also be explored by examining the values, beliefs and behaviours of an individual over their lifetime. Having a spiritual belief is thought to be helpful at reducing psychological distress and helping individuals find a sense of meaning in difficult situations.

Afterword

When we are faced with difficult decisions, many of which have no perfect solutions, we can feel powerless and despondent. Dealing with dementia can force many of these tricky choices upon us, but I hope the information contained in this book leaves you feeling better informed and helps you feel more assured and comfortable when responding to the various challenges involved.

Contrary to public opinion (at least, the views I have encountered in my work), there is much that can be done to protect yourself against dementia and/or delay its onset. It is important that we recognise these and act on them, ideally years before the condition usually develops. Likewise, there are numerous effective interventions and treatments that address the problems dementia can cause. I hope this book has illustrated this in an optimistic fashion. And even if there is nothing more we can do – we all have our limitations – then knowing this to be the case, and knowing that we are doing all we can, may be a source of comfort.

You are not alone in facing the difficulties that dementia creates. Many others are experiencing the same challenges. It is important that you reach out – whether to local support groups or family and friends – and not try to manage the situation all on your own. Having someone to talk to, with whom you can share your problems, can make all the difference between hope and despair. Educate yourself as best you can, and be guided by others who have gone through the same thing.

Acknowledgements

In preparing this book, I have become aware of the huge amount of past and ongoing research into dementia, both within Australia and internationally. I would like to acknowledge these efforts, without which much of the information in this book would have been impossible to impart.

I would also like to thank a number of people who have helped me produce this book, either through their direct input into its contents, their enthusiasm and facilitation of the publishing process, or their general support during the time it has taken to put it together.

Thank you firstly to my wife, Jennie, who, despite her own busy work as a radiologist, and the need to look after our three children, was unwavering in her forbearance as I regularly 'disappeared' into my writing, neglecting my husbandly and fatherly duties.

I'd also like to acknowledge Roger Hewitt, who provided valuable initial feedback about the book and who was instrumental in starting the chain that has eventually led to its publication. Many thanks also to Mario Pennisi and Madonna King for their advice and their critical role as further links in this chain.

I am also deeply indebted to Madonna Duffy, publishing director at University of Queensland Press, for her enthusiasm and recognition of the value of a book on dementia. Likewise, I am very grateful for the professionalism and personability of Julian Welch, who has edited this book into a much better product than the one initially delivered to him! Thanks also to Margot Lloyd for her efficient and helpful copyediting, and to Dr Matt Skalski for providing many of the illustrations.

I wish also to express my gratitude to all my peers and colleagues who took the time to go through the book and provide helpful tips. These include Dr Sarah Brooker, Dr John Barnett, Dr Bill Lukin, Dr Alan Coulthard, Fiona Coulthard and Rhonda Field. A special thank you also to Janice Rushworth for her forensic examination of the initial manuscript, and her advice on the importance of language choice.

I'd also like to thank my psychogeriatric colleagues in Brisbane, who have helped me improve my practice and provided invaluable insights into patient management throughout the years.

Finally, I'd like to acknowledge the many patients, family members and formal carers with whom I have had the pleasure of working over the last decade. They bring a wealth of knowledge and experience to the discussion of dementia, and I believe that I am a better doctor for having encountered them.

Appendix

General information and resources
Alzheimer's Disease International: www.alz.co.uk

Australia
Dementia Australia: www.dementia.org.au
National Dementia Helpline: 1800 100 500
Alzheimer's Association (Australia): www.alz.org/au/dementia-alzheimers-australia.asp
Queensland Brain Institute: https://qbi.uq.edu.au
Centre for Healthy Brain Ageing (CHeBA): https://cheba.unsw.edu.au
The Wicking Dementia Research and Education Centre: www.utas.edu.au/wicking
My Aged Care: www.myagedcare.gov.au

United Kingdom
Alzheimer's Society: www.alzheimers.org.uk

United States
Alzheimer's Association: www.alz.org
Dementia.org (Healthcare Brands): www.dementia.org

Exercise, nutrition and complex mental activity
Centre for Healthy Brain Ageing: https://cheba.unsw.edu.au/resources-for-individuals

Psychological illness

Beyond Blue: www.beyondblue.org.au

SANE Australia: www.sane.org

The Black Dog Institute: www.blackdoginstitute.org.au

Lifeline: 13 11 14

Assessment, BPSD and support

Dementia Support Australia (DSA) provides the services of the Dementia
Behaviour Management Advisory Service (DBMAS) and the Severe
Behavioural Response Team (SBRT): https://dementia.com.au;
phone, 1800 699 799

Incontinence

The Continence Foundation of Australia's National Continence Helpline:
1800 33 00 66; website: www.continence.org.au

Driving

Dementia Australia provides general information as well as links to the
driving licensing authorities in the various states and territories:
www.dementia.org.au/resources/dementia-and-driving

Respite care, funding and accommodation

My Aged Care: 1800 200 422; website, www.myagedcare.gov.au

Emergency respite care hotline: 1800 052 222 (during business hours) or
1800 059 059 (outside business hours)

Elder abuse

1800 ELDERHelp (national hotline to report elder abuse): 1800 353 374.
This number automatically transfers callers through to relevant phone
line services in their state or territory.

More information about these local services can be found on the website
of the Australian Institute of Family Studies – aifs.gov.au. Once on this
site, search for 'elder abuse support services'.

Advanced care directive and substitute decision-maker

Department of Health (Australia): www.health.gov.au/health-topics/
palliative-care/planning-your-palliative-care/advance-care-directive

Advance Care Planning Australia: www.advancecareplanning.org.au; phone: 1300 208 582

State and territory civil and administrative tribunals
- ACT Civil and Administrative Tribunal
  - www.acat.act.gov.au
  - 02 6207 1740
- New South Wales Civil and Administrative Tribunal
  - www.ncat.nsw.gov.au
  - 1300 006 228
- Northern Territory Civil and Administrative Tribunal (NTCAT)
  - ntcat.nt.gov.au
  - 1800 604 622
- Queensland Civil and Administrative Tribunal (QCAT)
  - www.qcat.qld.gov.au
  - 1300 753 228
- South Australian Civil and Administrative Tribunal (SACAT)
  - www.sacat.sa.gov.au
  - 1800 723 767
- Tasmanian Guardianship and Administrative Board
  - www.guardianship.tas.gov.au
  - 1300 799 625
- Victorian Civil and Administrative Tribunal (VCAT)
  - www.vcat.vic.gov.au
  - 1300 018 228
- Western Australian State Administrative Tribunal (SAT)
  - www.sat.justice.wa.gov.au
  - 1300 306 017

Public trustees
- Public Trustee (Australian Capital Territory)
  - www.publictrustee.act.gov.au
  - 02 6207 9800
- NSW Trustee and Guardian
  - www.tag.nsw.gov.au
  - 1300 364 103

- Public Trustee (Northern Territory)
  - nt.gov.au/law/processes/about–public–trustee
  - 1800 517 223
- Public Trustee (Queensland)
  - www.pt.qld.gov.au
  - 1300 360 044
- Public Trustee (South Australia)
  - www.publictrustee.sa.gov.au
  - 1800 673 119
- Public Trustee (Tasmania)
  - www.publictrustee.tas.gov.au
  - 1800 068 784
- State Trustees (Victoria)
  - www.statetrustees.com.au
  - 1300 138 672
- Public Trustee (Western Australia)
  - www.publictrustee.wa.gov.au
  - 1300 746 212

Sources

General

Alzheimer's Disease International

Dementia Australia

Alzheimer's Association (Australia)

Queensland Brain Institute

Centre for Healthy Brain Ageing (CHeBA)

The Wicking Dementia Research and Education Centre

My Aged Care

Alzheimer's Society (UK)

Alzheimer's Association (US)

Alzheimer's Association (Canada)

Cochranelibrary.com

American Psychiatric Association, *Diagnostic and Statistical Manual of Mental Disorders* (fifth edition)

Chapter 1: How the Brain Functions

B. Dubuc, *The Brain from Top to Bottom* (website), https://thebrain.mcgill.ca.

E.A. Maguire et al., 'Navigation-related structural change in the hippocampi of taxi drivers', *Proceedings of the National Academy of Sciences of the United States of America*, vol. 97, no. 8, pp. 4398–403, 2000.

M.E. Raichle & D.A. Gusnard, 'Appraising the brain's energy budget', *PNAS*, vol. 99, no. 16, pp. 10237–39, 2002.

University of Queensland, *Queensland Brain Institute* (website), https://qbi.uq.edu.au.

Chapter 2: Normal Ageing and Cognition

Chen, Y. et al., 'Arterial stiffness and stroke: De-stiffening strategy, a therapeutic target for stroke', *Stroke and Vascular Neurology*, vol. 2, no. 2, 2017.

C.N. Harada et al., 'Normal cognitive aging', *Clinical Geriatric Medicine*, vol. 29, no. 4, pp. 737–52, 2013.

B. Jani & C. Rajkumar, 'Ageing and vascular ageing', *Postgraduate Medical Journal*, vol. 82, no. 968, pp. 357–62, 2006.

R. Peters, 'Ageing and the brain', *Postgraduate Medical Journal*, vol. 82, no. 964, pp. 84–8, 2006.

L. Svennerholm et al., 'Changes in weight and compositions of major membrane components of human brain during the span of adult human life of Swedes', *Acta Neuropathologica*, vol. 94, no. 4, pp. 345–52, 1997.

Chapter 3: Preventing Cognitive Decline

ACHIEVE Healthy Aging, *Aging and Cognitive Health Evaluation in Elders Study*, www.achievestudy.org.

Alzheimer's Australia NSW, *The Benefits of Physical Activity and Exercise for People Living with Dementia*, Discussion Paper 11, November 2014, www.dementia.org.au/sites/default/files/NSW/documents/AANSW_DiscussionPaper11.pdf.

H. Amieva et al., 'Self-reported hearing loss, hearing aids, and cognitive decline in elderly adults: A 25-year study', *Journal of the American Geriatrics Society*, vol. 63, no. 10, pp. 2099–104, 2015.

Australian Institute of Health and Welfare, *Impact of Physical Inactivity as a Risk Factor for Chronic Conditions: Australian Burden of Disease*, report released 22 November 2017.

Centre for Healthy Brain Ageing, *Maintain Your Brain* (website), www.maintainyourbrain.org.

L.J. Cherian et al., 'Abstract 152: Dietary patterns associated with slower cognitive decline post stroke', vol. 49, supp. 1, 2018.

V.C. Crooks et al., 'Social network, cognitive function, and dementia incidence among elderly women', *American Journal of Public Health*, vol. 98, no.7, pp. 1221–27, 2008.

R. de Cabo & Mark P. Mattson, 'Effects of intermittent fasting on health, aging, and disease', *New England Journal of Medicine*, no. 381, pp. 2541–51, 2019.

Dementia Australia, 'What you eat and drink and your brain' (fact sheet), 2015 [2006], www.dementia.org.au/sites/default/files/helpsheets/Help sheet-DementiaQandA07-WhatYouEatAndDrinkAndYourBrain_ english.pdf.

K. Ebrahimi et al., 'Physical activity and beta-amyloid pathology in Alzheimer's disease: A sound mind in a sound body', *EXCLI Journal*, vol. 16, pp. 959–72, 2017.

R.F. Gottesman et al., 'Association between midlife vascular risk factors and estimated brain amyloid deposition', *JAMA*, vol. 317, no. 14, pp. 1443–50, 2017.

F. Herold et al., 'Functional and/or structural brain changes in response to resistance exercises and resistance training lead to cognitive improvements – a systematic review', *European Review of Aging and Physical Activity*, vol. 16, article no. 10, 2019.

M.K. Jedrziewski et al., 'The impact of exercise, cognitive activities, and socialization on cognitive function: Results from the National Long-Term Care Survey', *American Journal of Alzheimer's Disease & Other Dementias*, vol. 29, no. 4, pp. 372–8, 2014.

J.S. Kuiper et al., 'Social relationships and risk of dementia: A systematic review and meta-analysis of longitudinal cohort studies', *Aging Research Reviews*, vol. 22, pp. 39–57, 2015.

E.B. Larson, 'Exercise is associated with reduced risk for incident dementia among persons 65 years of age and older', *Annals of Internal Medicine*, vol. 144, no. 2, pp. 73–81, 2006.

N.T. Lautenschlager et al., 'Effect of physical activity on cognitive function in older adults at risk for Alzheimer's disease: A randomized trial', *JAMA*, vol. 300, no. 9, pp. 1027–37, 2008.

L. Mandolesi et al., 'Effects of physical exercise on cognitive functioning and wellbeing: Biological and psychological benefits', *Frontiers in Psychology*, vol. 9, p. 509, 2018.

Mayo Clinic, 'Mediterranean diet: A heart-healthy eating plan', 21 June 2019, www.mayoclinic.org/healthy-lifestyle/nutrition-and-healthy-eating/in-depth/mediterranean-diet/art-20047801.

N. McKeehan, 'Paleo and ketogenic diets on the brain', *Cognitive Vitality*, 9 August 2016, www.alzdiscovery.org/cognitive-vitality/blog/paleo-and-keto-on-the-brain.

N. McKeehan, 'Is exercise bad for dementia patients? A new study makes odd claim', *Cognitive Vitality*, 5 June 2018, www.alzdiscovery.org/cognitive-vitality/blog/is-exercise-bad-for-dementia-patients.

O. Mesarwi et al., 'Sleep disorders and the development of insulin resistance and obesity', *Endocrinology and Metabolism Clinics of North America*, vol. 42, no. 3, pp. 617–34, 2013.

M.C. Morris et al., 'MIND diet slows cognitive decline with aging', *Alzheimer's & Dementia*, vol. 11, no. 9, pp. 1015–22, 2015.

I. Mosnier et al., 'Improvement of cognitive function after cochlear implantation in elderly patients', JAMA Otolaryngology – Head & Neck Surgery, vol. 141, no. 5, pp. 442–50, 2015.

Tiia Ngandu et al., 'A 2 year multidomain intervention of diet, exercise, cognitive training, and vascular risk monitoring versus control to prevent cognitive decline in at-risk elderly people (FINGER): A randomised controlled trial', *The Lancet*, vol. 385, no. 9984, pp. 2255–63, 2015.

S. Norton et al., 'Potential for primary prevention of Alzheimer's disease: An analysis of population-based data', *The Lancet Neurology*, vol. 13, no. 8, pp. 788–94, 2014.

R. Penninkilampi et al., 'The association between social engagement, loneliness, and risk of dementia: A systematic review and meta-analysis', *Journal of Alzheimer's Disease*, vol. 66, no. 4, pp. 1619–33, 2018.

G. Ravaglia et al., 'Physical activity and dementia risk in the elderly: Findings from a prospective Italian study', *Neurology*, vol. 70, no. 19, pt 2, pp. 1786–94, 2008.

A. Sauer, 'The link between vascular disease and Alzheimer's', *Alzheimers. net*, 24 May 2017, www.alzheimers.net/05-24-17-vascular-disease-dementia.

A. Solomon et al., 'Midlife serum cholesterol and increased risk of Alzheimer's and vascular dementia three decades later', *Dementia and Geriatric Cognitive Disorders*, vol. 28, no. 1, pp. 75–80, 2009.

S.F. Sorrells et al., 'Human hippocampal neurogenesis drops sharply in children to undetectable levels in adults', *Nature*, vol. 555, pp. 377–81, 2018.

S.J. Spencer, 'Food for thought: How nutrition impacts cognition and emotion', *NPJ Science of Food*, vol. 1, no. 7, 2017.

T. Tanaka et al., 'Adherence to a Mediterranean diet protects from cognitive decline in the Invecchiare in Chianti Study of Aging', *Nutrients*, vol. 10, no. 12, 2007, 2018.

M.J. Valenzuela & P. Sachdev, 'Brain reserve and dementia: A systematic review', *Psychological Medicine*, vol. 36, no. 4, pp. 441–54, 2006.

M.J. Valenzuela et al., 'Complex mental activity and the aging brain: Molecular, cellular and cortical network mechanisms', *Brain Research Reviews*, vol. 56, pp. 198–213, 2007.

R.S. Wilson et al., 'Loneliness and risk of Alzheimer disease', *Archives of General Psychiatry*, vol. 64, no. 2, pp. 234–40, 2007.

D. Włodarek, 'Role of ketogenic diets in neurodegenerative diseases (Alzheimer's disease and Parkinson's disease)', *Nutrients*, vol. 11, no. 1, p. 169, 2019.

D. Zhen et al., 'Physical activity can improve cognition in patients with Alzheimer's disease: A systematic review and meta-analysis of randomized controlled trials', *Clinical Interventions in Aging*, vol. 13, pp. 1593–1603, 2018.

F. Zheng et al., 'HbA$_{1c}$, diabetes and cognitive decline: The English Longitudinal Study of Ageing', *Diabetologia*, vol. 61, no. 4, pp. 839–48, 2018.

Chapter 4: Supplements and Vitamins in Cognition

Alcohol and Drug Foundation, 'What is caffeine?', 5 June 2020, https://adf.org.au/drug-facts/caffeine.

Alzheimer's Society (UK), 'Caffeine and dementia', www.alzheimers.org.uk/about-dementia/risk-factors-and-prevention/caffeine-and-dementia.

G. Arendash & C. Cao, 'Caffeine and coffee as therapeutics against Alzheimer's disease', *Journal of Alzheimer's Disease*, vol. 20, supp. 1, pp. S117–26, 2010.

R. Baeta-Corral et al., 'Long-term treatment with low-dose caffeine worsens BPSD-like profile in 3xTg-AD mice model of Alzheimer's disease and affects mice with normal aging', *Frontiers in Pharmacology*, vol. 9, p. 79, 2018.

S.K. Bhattacharya et al., 'Antioxidant activity of Bacopa monniera in rat frontal cortex, striatum and hippocampus', *Phytotherapy Research*, vol. 14, no. 3, pp. 174–9, 2000.

M. Burckhardt et al., 'Omega-3 fatty acids for the treatment of dementia', *The Cochrane Database of Systematic Reviews*, issue 4, article no. CD009002, 2016.

K.S. Chaudhari, 'Neurocognitive effect of nootropic drug brahmi (Bacopa monnieri) in Alzheimer's disease', *Annals of Neurosciences*, vol. 24, no. 2, pp. 111–22, 2017.

Dementia Australia, 'Souvenaid: A dietary treatment for mild Alzheimer's disease' (fact sheet), 2019 [2013], www.dementia.org.au/sites/default/files/helpsheets/Helpsheet-DementiaQandA23-Souvenaid_english.pdf.

M.H. Eskelinen & M. Kivipelto, 'Caffeine as a protective factor in dementia and Alzheimer's disease', *Journal of Alzheimer's Disease*, vol. 20, supp. 1, pp. S167–74, 2010.

N. Farina et al., 'The use of vitamin E in the treatment of mild cognitive impairment and Alzheimer's disease (AD)', *The Cochrane Database of Systematic Reviews*, issue 4, article no. CD002854, 2017.

J. Graff-Radford, 'Vitamin D: Can it prevent Alzheimer's dementia?', *Mayo Clinic*, 23 April 2019, www.mayoclinic.org/diseases-conditions/alzheimers-disease/expert-answers/vitamin-d-alzheimers/faq-20111272.

Y. Hara, 'New debate on hormone replacement therapy and dementia risk', *Cognitive Vitality*, 22 March 2017, www.alzdiscovery.org/cognitive-vitality/blog/new-debate-on-hormone-replacement-therapy-and-dementia-risk.

Institute of Medicine (US) Committee on Military Nutrition Research, *Caffeine for the Sustainment of Mental Task Performance: Formulations for military operations*. Washington DC: National Academies Press, 2001.

D. Jaturapatporn et al., 'Aspirin, steroidal and non-steroidal anti-inflammatory drugs for the treatment of Alzheimer's disease', *The Cochrane Database of Systematic Reviews*, issue 2, article no. CD006378, 2012.

T.J. Littlejohns et al., 'Vitamin D and the risk of dementia and Alzheimer disease', *Neurology*, vol. 83, no. 10, pp. 920–8, 2014.

M. Mazza et al., 'Ginkgo biloba and donepezil: A comparison in the treatment of Alzheimer's dementia in a randomized placebo-controlled double-blind study', *European Journal of Neurology*, vol. 13, no. 9, pp. 981–5, 2006.

J. McCleery et al., 'Vitamin and mineral supplementation for preventing dementia or delaying cognitive decline in people with mild cognitive impairment', *The Cochrane Database of Systematic Reviews*, issue 11, article no. CD011905, 2018.

T.M. McLellan et al., 'A review of caffeine's effects on cognitive, physical and occupational performance', *Neuroscience & Biobehavioral Reviews*, vol. 71, pp. 294–312, 2016.

N.M. Nasab et al., 'Efficacy of rivastigmine in comparison to ginkgo for treating Alzheimer's dementia', *The Journal of the Pakistan Medical Association*, vol. 62, no. 7, pp. 677–80, 2012.

M.P. Pase et al., 'The cognitive-enhancing effects of Bacopa monnieri: A systematic review of randomized, controlled human clinical trials', Journal of Alternative and Complementary Medicine, vol. 18, no. 7, pp. 647–52, 2012.

Y. Qiuju et al., 'Effects of Ginkgo biloba on dementia: An overview of systematic reviews', *Journal of Ethnopharmacology*, vol. 195, pp. 1–9, 2017.

Queensland Brain Institute, 'Vitamin D deficiency a risk factor for cognitive decline and dementia', 12 December 2018, https://qbi.uq.edu.au/article/2018/12/vitamin-d-deficiency-risk-factor-cognitive-decline-and-dementia.

S. Roodenrys et al., 'Chronic effects of brahmi (Bacopa monnieri) on human memory', *Neuropsychopharmacology*, vol. 27, pp. 279–81, 2002.

H. Savolainen-Peltonen et al., 'Use of postmenopausal hormone therapy and risk of Alzheimer's disease in Finland: Nationwide case-control study', *BMJ*, vol. 364, 1665, 2019.

R.H. Shmerling, 'The latest scoop on the health benefits of coffee', *Harvard Health Publishing*, 25 September 2017, www.health.harvard.edu/blog/the-latest-scoop-on-the-health-benefits-of-coffee-2017092512429.

H. Soininen et al., '24-month intervention with a specific multinutrient in people with prodromal Alzheimer's disease (LipiDiDiet): A randomised, double-blind, controlled trial', *The Lancet Neurology*, vol. 16, no. 12, pp. 965–75, 2017.

G.W. Small et al., 'Memory and brain amyloid and tau effects of a bioavailable form of curcumin in non-demented adults: A double-blind, placebo-controlled 18-month trial', *The American Journal of Geriatric Psychiatry*, vol. 26, no. 3, pp. 266–77, 2018.

S.J. Spencer, 'Food for thought: How nutrition impacts cognition and emotion', *NPJ Science of Food*, vol. 1, no. 7, 2017.

E. Sydenham et al., 'Omega 3 fatty acid for the prevention of cognitive decline and dementia', *The Cochrane Database of Systematic Reviews*, issue 6, article no. CD005379, 2012.

The Brain from Top to Bottom, 'Caffeine', https://thebrain.mcgill.ca/flash/i/i_03/i_03_m/i_03_m_par/i_03_m_par_cafeine.html.

D. Zhen et al., 'Physical activity can improve cognition in patients with Alzheimer's disease: A systematic review and meta-analysis of randomized controlled trials', *Clinical Interventions in Aging*, vol. 13, pp. 1593–1603, 2018.

Chapter 5: Reversible Cognitive Impairment

S. Ouanes & J. Popp, 'High cortisol and the risk of dementia and Alzheimer's disease: A review of the literature', *Frontiers in Aging Neuroscience*, vol. 11, article no. 43, 2019.

B. Solé et al., 'Cognitive impairment in bipolar disorder: Treatment and prevention strategies', *International Journal of Neuropsychopharmacology*, vol. 20, no. 8, pp. 670–80, 2017.

Chapter 6: More than Ageing, but Not Dementia

K.M. Broadhouse et al., 'Hippocampal plasticity underpins long-term cognitive gains from resistance exercise in MCI', *NeuroImage: Clinical*, vol. 25, article 102182, 2020.

M. Butler et al., 'Does cognitive training prevent cognitive decline? A systematic review', *Annals of Internal Medicine*, vol. 168, no. 1, pp. 63–8, 2018.

Cedars Sinai, 'Subjective cognitive impairment (SCI)', 2019, www.cedars-sinai.edu/Patients/Health-Conditions/Subjective-Cognitive-Impairment-SCI.aspx.

A. Espinosa et al., 'A longitudinal follow-up of 550 mild cognitive impairment patients: Evidence for large conversion to dementia rates and detection of major risk factors involved', *Journal of Alzheimer's Disease*, vol. 34, pp. 769–80, 2013.

C. Jonker et al., 'Are memory complaints predictive for dementia? A review of clinical and population-based studies', *International Journal of Geriatric Psychiatry*, vol. 15, no. 11, pp. 983–91, 2000.

A.J. Mitchell et al., 'Risk of dementia and mild cognitive impairment in older people with subjective memory complaints: Meta-analysis', *Acta Psychiatrica Scandinavica*, vol. 130, no. 6, pp. 439–51, 2014.

A. Okello et al., 'Conversion of amyloid positive and negative MCI to AD over 3 years: An ^{11}C-PIB PET study', *Neurology*, vol. 73, no. 10, pp. 754–60, 2009.

T.C. Russ & J.R. Morling, 'Cholinesterase inhibitors for mild cognitive impairment', *The Cochrane Database of Systematic Reviews*, issue 9, article no. CD009132, 2012.

L. Xiao-Xue & L. Zheng, 'The impact of anxiety on the progression of mild cognitive impairment to dementia in Chinese and English data bases: A systematic review and meta-analysis', *International Journal of Geriatric Psychiatry*, vol. 33, no. 1, pp. 131–40, 2018.

B.S. Ye et al., 'Longitudinal outcomes of amyloid positive versus negative amnestic mild cognitive impairments: A three-year longitudinal study', *Scientific Reports*, vol. 8, article no. 5557, 2018.

Chapter 7: Dementia Defined

R.J. Harvey et al., 'The prevalence and causes of dementia in people under the age of 65 years', *Journal of Neurology, Neurosurgery & Psychiatry*, vol. 74, pp. 1206–9, 2003.

A. Lobo et al., 'Prevalence of dementia and major subtypes in Europe: A collaborative study of population-based cohorts. Neurologic diseases in the elderly research group', *Neurology*, vol. 54, no. 11, supp. 5, pp. S4–9, 2000.

W.M. van der Flier & P. Scheltens, 'Epidemiology and risk factors of dementia', *Journal of Neurology, Neurosurgery & Psychiatry*, vol. 76, pp. v2–v7, 2005.

Young Dementia UK, 'Young onset dementia facts & figures', *Young Dementia UK* (website), 2020, www.youngdementiauk.org/young-onset-dementia-facts-figures.

Chapter 8: Alzheimer's Disease and Vascular Dementia

F. Alasmari et al., 'Neuroinflammatory cytokines induce amyloid beta neurotoxicity through modulating amyloid precursor protein levels/metabolism', BioMed Research International, vol. 2018, article ID 3087475.

A. Altmann et al., 'Sex modifies the APOE-related risk of developing Alzheimer disease', *Annals of Neurology*, vol. 75, no. 4, pp. 563–73, 2014.

Alzheimer's Research UK, 'Genes and dementia', 2018, www.alzheimersresearchuk.org/dementia-information/genes-and-dementia.

Alzheimer's Society, 'Risk factors for dementia' (fact sheet), 2017, www.alzheimers.org.uk/sites/default/files/pdf/factsheet_risk_factors_for_dementia.pdf.

Alzheimer's Society, 'Symptoms of Alzheimer's disease', 2020, www.alzheimers.org.uk/about-dementia/types-dementia/alzheimers-disease-symptoms.

S. Askarova et al., 'The links between the gut microbiome, aging, modern lifestyle and Alzheimer's disease', *Front Cell Infect Microbiol.*, 2020.

L. Bertram et al., 'Systematic meta-analyses of Alzheimer disease genetic association studies: The AlzGene database', *Nature Genetics*, vol. 39, pp. 17–23, 2007.

J.C. Breitner et al., 'Familial aggregation in Alzheimer's disease: Comparison of risk among relatives of early- and late-onset cases, and among male and female relatives in successive generations', *Neurology*, vol. 38, no. 2, pp. 207–12, 1988.

Q. Chengxuan et al., 'Epidemiology of Alzheimer's disease: Occurrence, determinants, and strategies toward intervention', *Dialogues in Clinical Neuroscience*, vol. 11, no. 2, pp. 111–28, 2009.

S. Choi et al., 'Association of chronic periodontitis on Alzheimer's disease or vascular dementia', *J. Am. Geriatr. Soc.*, 2019.

J.L. Cummings et al., 'International work group criteria for the diagnosis of Alzheimer disease', *The Medical Clinics of North America*, vol. 97, no. 3, pp. 363–8, 2013.

Dementia Australia, 'Anaesthesia for older people and people with dementia' (fact sheet), 2018 [2007], www.dementia.org.au/sites/default/files/helpsheets/Helpsheet-DementiaQandA20-Anaethesia_english.pdf.

G.A. Edwards III et al., 'Modifiable risk factors for Alzheimer's disease', *Frontiers in Aging Neuroscience*, vol. 11, article no. 146, 2019.

L.S.S. Ferreira et al., 'Insulin resistance in Alzheimer's disease', *Front. Neurosci.*, 2018.

T. Fulop et al., 'Can an infection hypothesis explain the beta amyloid hypothesis of Alzheimer's disease?', *Frontiers in Aging Neuroscience*, vol. 10, article no. 224, 2018.

E. Grober et al., 'Free and cued selective reminding distinguishes Alzheimer's disease from vascular dementia', *Journal of the American Geriatrics Society*, vol. 56, no. 5, pp. 944–6, 2008.

N.A. Jessen, et al., 'The glymphatic system: A beginner's guide', *Neurochemical Research*, vol. 40, no. 12, pp. 2583–99, 2015.

D. Kellar & S. Craft, 'Brain insulin resistance in Alzheimer's disease and related disorders: Mechanisms and therapeutic approaches', *The Lancet*, vol. 19, no. 9, pp. 758–66, 2020.

R. La Joie et al., 'Prospective longitudinal atrophy in Alzheimer's disease correlates with the intensity and topography of baseline tau-PET', *Science Translational Medicine*, vol. 12, no. 524, 2020.

T. Laukkanen et al., 'Sauna bathing is inversely associated with dementia and Alzheimer's disease in middle-aged Finnish men', *Age and Ageing*, vol. 46, no. 2, pp. 245–9, 2017.

S.Q. Li et al., 'Dementia prevalence and incidence among the Indigenous and non-Indigenous populations of the Northern Territory', *Medical Journal of Australia*, vol. 200, no. 8, pp. 465–9, 2014.

G. Livingston et al., 'Dementia prevention, intervention, and care', *The Lancet*, vol. 390, issue 10113, pp. 2673–734, 2017.

S. Makin, 'The amyloid hypothesis on trial', *Nature*, vol. 559, pp. S4–S7, 2018.

G.M. McKhann et al., 'The diagnosis of dementia due to Alzheimer's disease: Recommendations from the National Institute on Aging-Alzheimer's Association workgroups on diagnostic guidelines for Alzheimer's disease', *Alzheimer's and Dementia*, vol. 7, no. 3, pp. 263–9, 2011.

Multimedia Neuroscience Education Project, 'IA5. Clinical application: Acetylcholine and Alzheimer's disease', https://web.williams.edu/imput/synapse/pages/IA5.html.

M. Musicco et al., 'Predictors of progression of cognitive decline in Alzheimer's disease: The role of vascular and sociodemographic factors', *Journal of Neurology*, vol. 256, no. 8, pp. 1288–95, 2009.

National Institute on Aging, 'Alzheimer's disease genetics fact sheet', 2019, www.nia.nih.gov/health/alzheimers-disease-genetics-fact-sheet.

National Institute of Neurological Disorders and Stroke, 'Binswanger's disease information page', 2019, www.ninds.nih.gov/Disorders/All-Disorders/Binswangers-Disease-Information-Page.

S. Palmqvist et al., 'Discriminative accuracy of plasma phospho-tau217 for Alzheimer disease vs other neurodegenerative disorders', *JAMA*, published online, 28 July 2020.

S. Salimi et al., 'Can visuospatial measures improve the diagnosis of Alzheimer's disease?', *Alzheimer's & Dementia*, vol. 10, pp. 66–74, 2018.

E. Shokri-Kojori et al., 'β-Amyloid accumulation in the human brain after one night of sleep deprivation', *PNAS*, vol. 115, no. 17, pp. 4483–8, 2018.

A.D. Smith et al., 'Homocysteine and dementia: An international consensus statement', *Journal of Alzheimer's Disease*, vol. 62, no. 2, pp. 561–70, 2018.

K. Smith et al., 'High prevalence of dementia and cognitive impairment in Indigenous Australians', *Neurology*, vol. 71, no. 19, pp. 1470–3, 2008.

L. Teri et al., 'Cognitive decline in Alzheimer's disease: A longitudinal investigation of risk factors for accelerated decline', *The Journals of Gerontology. Series A, Biological Sciences and Medical Sciences*, vol 50A, no. 1, pp. M49–55, 1995.

W.M. van der Flier & P. Scheltens, 'Epidemiology and risk factors of dementia', *Journal of Neurology, Neurosurgery & Psychiatry*, vol. 76, pp. v2–v7, 2005.

D. Xiaoguang et al., 'Alzheimer's disease hypothesis and related therapies', *Translational Neurodegeneration*, vol. 7, p. 2, 2018.

W. Yuchi et al., 'Road proximity, air pollution, noise, green space and neurologic disease incidence: A population-based cohort study', *Environmental Health*, vol. 19, article no. 8, 2020.

Chapter 9: Frontotemporal, Alcohol-related and Subcortical Dementias

Alzheimer's Association, 'Normal pressure hydrocephalus', 2020, www. alz.org/alzheimers-dementia/what-is-dementia/types-of-dementia/ normal-pressure-hydrocephalus.

Alzheimer's Association, 'Parkinson's disease dementia', 2020, www.alz. org/alzheimers-dementia/what-is-dementia/types-of-dementia/ parkinson-s-disease-dementia.

Alzheimer's Society, 'Alcohol and dementia', 2020, www.alzheimers.org. uk/about-dementia/risk-factors-and-prevention/alcohol.

Better Health Channel, 'Alcohol related brain impairment – memory loss', 2015, www.betterhealth.vic.gov.au/health/conditionsandtreatments/ alcohol-related-brain-impairment-memory-loss.

Brain Foundation, 'Progressive supranuclear palsy', 2020, https:// brainfoundation.org.au/disorders/progressive-supranuclear-palsy.

A. Cagnin et al., 'Sleep-wake profile in dementia with Lewy bodies, Alzheimer's disease, and normal aging', *Journal of Alzheimer's Disease*, vol. 55, no. 4, pp. 1529–36, 2017.

K. Cherry, 'Does drinking alcohol kill brain cells?', *Very Well Mind*, 16 May

2020, www.verywellmind.com/does-drinking-alcohol-really-kill-brain-cells-2794887.

J.L. Cummings & D.F. Benson, 'Subcortical dementia. Review of an emerging concept', *Archives of Neurology*, vol. 41, no. 8, pp. 874–9, 1984.

Dementia Australia, 'HIV associated dementia', 2020, www.dementia.org.au/about-dementia/types-of-dementia/aids-related-dementia.

Dementia Australia, 'Lewy body disease', 2020, www.dementia.org.au/about-dementia/types-of-dementia/lewy-body-disease.

E. Devenney et al., 'The behavioural variant frontotemporal dementia phenocopy syndrome is a distinct entity – evidence from a longitudinal study', *BMC Neurology*, vol. 18, article no. 56, 2018.

E.W. Dolan, 'Problematic alcohol use linked to reduced hippocampal volume', *PsyPost*, 9 December 2017, www.psypost.org/2017/12/problematic-alcohol-use-linked-reduced-hippocampal-volume-50354.

R.L. Hamilton, 'Lewy bodies in Alzheimer's disease: A neuropathological review of 145 cases using alpha-synuclein immunohistochemistry', *Brain Pathology*, vol. 10, no. 3, pp. 378–84, 2000.

D.B. Hogan et al. 'The prevalence and incidence of frontotemporal dementia: A systematic review', *Canadian Journal of Neurological Sciences*, vol. 43, supp. 1, pp. S96–S109, 2016.

S.J. Huber & G.W. Paulson, 'The concept of subcortical dementia', *The American Journal of Psychiatry*, vol. 142, no. 11, pp. 1312–7, 1985.

T. Järvenpää et al., 'Binge drinking in midlife and dementia risk', *Epidemiology*, vol. 16, no. 6, pp. 766–71, 2005.

Johns Hopkins Medicine, 'HIV and dementia', 2020, www.hopkinsmedicine.org/health/conditions-and-diseases/hiv-and-aids/hiv-and-dementia.

J. Malm et al., 'Influence of comorbidities in idiopathic normal pressure hydrocephalus – research and clinical care. A report of the ISHCSF task force on comorbidities in INPH', *Fluids and Barriers of the CNS*, vol. 10, no. 1, p. 22, 2013.

Medline Plus, 'Wernicke-Korsakoff syndrome', 2020, https://medlineplus.gov/ency/article/000771.htm.

M. Mizuko, 'Symptoms of Aphasia', www.d.umn.edu/~mmizuko/2230/sym.htm.

National Health and Medical Research Council, *Draft Australian Guidelines to Reduce Health Risks from Drinking Alcohol*, December 2019, www.nhmrc.gov.au/sites/default/files/documents/attachments/draft-aus-guidelines-reduce-health-risks-alcohol.pdf.

National Institute of Neurological Disorders and Stroke, 'Corticobasal degeneration information page', 2019, www.ninds.nih.gov/Disorders/All-Disorders/Corticobasal-Degeneration-Information-Page.

L.M. Oliveira et al., 'Cognitive dysfunction in corticobasal degeneration', *Arquivos de Neuropsiquiatria*, vol. 75, no. 8, pp. 570–9, 2017.

D.W. Oslin & M.S. Cary, 'Alcohol-related dementia: Validation of diagnostic criteria', *American Journal of Geriatric Psychiatry*, vol. 11, no. 4, pp. 441–7, 2003.

Parkinson's Victoria, 'Dementia and cognitive change', n.d., www.parkinsonsvic.org.au/parkinsons-and-you/dementia-and-cognitive-change.

Physiopedia, 'Lewy body disease', 2020, www.physio-pedia.com/Lewy_Body_Disease.

Queensland Brain Institute, 'Genetic risk factors for dementia', 2019, https://qbi.uq.edu.au/brain/dementia/genetic-risk-factors-dementia.

N.J. Ridley et al., 'Alcohol-related dementia: An update of the evidence', *Alzheimer's Research & Therapy*, vol. 5, no. 1, p. 3, 2013.

H.A. Ring & J. Serra-Mestres, 'Neuropsychiatry of the basal ganglia', *Journal of Neurology, Neurosurgery & Psychiatry*, vol. 72, pp. 12–21, 2002.

M.J. Schneck, 'Normal pressure hydrocephalus clinical presentation', *Medscape*, 19 October 2018, https://emedicine.medscape.com/article/1150924-clinical.

R.M. Shmerling, 'Sorting out the health effects of alcohol', *Harvard Health Publishing*, 6 August 2018, www.health.harvard.edu/blog/sorting-out-the-health-effects-of-alcohol-2018080614427.

M.A. Turner et al., 'Subcortical dementia', *British Journal of Psychiatry*, vol. 180, no. 2, pp. 148–51, 2002.

K.J. Woodburn & E.C. Johnstone, 'Early-onset dementia in Lothian, Scotland: An analysis of clinical features and patterns of decline', *Health Bulletin*, vol. 57, no. 6, pp. 384–92, 1999.

W. Xu et al., 'Alcohol consumption and dementia risk: A dose-response meta-analysis of prospective studies', *European Journal of Epidemiology*, vol. 32, no. 1, pp. 31–42, 2017.

Chapter 11: Medical History

D.E. Barnes et al., 'Midlife vs late-life depressive symptoms and risk of dementia: Differential effects for Alzheimer disease and vascular dementia', *Archives of General Psychiatry*, vol. 69, no. 5, pp. 493–8, 2012.

J.-M. Bugnicourt et al., 'Cognitive disorders and dementia in CKD: The neglected kidney-brain axis', *Journal of the American Society of Nephrology*, vol. 24, no. 3, pp. 353–63, 2013.

C. Chu et al., 'Use of statins and the risk of dementia and mild cognitive impairment: A systematic review and meta-analysis', *Scientific Reports*, vol. 8, article no. 5804, 2018.

R. Devere, 'Dementia insights: Cognitive consequences of perimenopause', *Practical Neurology*, May 2019, https://practicalneurology.com/articles/2019-may/dementia-insights-cognitive-consequences-ofperi menopause.

M.A. Evans & B.A. Golomb, 'Statin-associated adverse cognitive effects: Survey results from 171 patients', *Pharmacotherapy*, vol. 29, no. 7, pp. 800–11, 2009.

Harvard Health Publishing, 'Perimenopause: Rocky road to menopause', 14 April 2020 [2009], www.health.harvard.edu/womens-health/perimenopause-rocky-road-to-menopause.

B.J. Hasselbalch et al., 'Cognitive deficits in the remitted state of unipolar depressive disorder', *Neuropsychology*, vol. 26, no. 5, pp. 642–51, 2012.

H. Kang et al., 'Decreased expression of synapse-related genes and loss of synapses in major depressive disorder', *Nature Medicine*, vol. 18, pp. 1413–7, 2012.

B. McGuinness et al., 'Statins for the prevention of dementia', *The Cochrane Database of Systematic Reviews*, issue 1, article no. CD003160, 2016.

Mental Illness Policy Org, 'Cognitive impairment: A major problem for individuals with schizophrenia and bipolar disorder', n.d., https://mentalillnesspolicy.org/medical/cognitive-impairment.html.

M.W. Moyer, 'It's not dementia, it's your heart medication: Cholesterol drugs and memory', *Scientific American*, 1 September 2010, www.scientificamerican.com/article/its-not-dementia-its-your-heart-medication.

M.F. Muldoon et al., 'Effects of lovastatin on cognitive function and psychological wellbeing', *American Journal of Medicine*, vol. 108, pp. 538–47, 2000.

M.F. Muldoon et al., 'Randomized trial of the effects of simvastatin on cognitive functioning in hypercholesterolemic adults', *American Journal of Medicine*, vol. 117, no. 11, pp. 823–9, 2004.

J.W. Murrough et al., 'Cognitive dysfunction in depression: Neurocircuitry and new therapeutic strategies', *Neurobiology of Learning and Memory*, vol. 96, no. 4, pp. 553–63, 2011.

R.H. Pietrzak et al., 'Plasma cortisol, brain amyloid-β, and cognitive decline in preclinical Alzheimer's disease: A 6-year prospective cohort study', *Biological Psychiatry CNNI*, vol. 2, no. 1, pp. 45–52, 2017.

B.G. Schultz et al., 'The role of statins in both cognitive impairment and protection against dementia: A tale of two mechanisms', *Translational Neurodegeneration*, vol. 7, no. 5, 2018.

K.J. Swiger, 'Statins and cognition: A systematic review and meta-analysis of short- and long-term cognitive effects', *Mayo Clinic Proceedings*, vol. 88, no. 11, pp. 1213–21, 2013.

J. Verghese et al., 'Abnormality of gait as a predictor of non-Alzheimer's dementia', *The New England Journal of Medicine*, vol. 347, pp. 1761–8, 2002.

Y. Yang et al., 'Cognitive impairment in generalized anxiety disorder revealed by event-related potential N270', *Neuropsychiatric Disease and Treatment*, vol. 11, pp. 1405–11, 2015.

Chapter 12: Physical Examination and Cognitive Testing

J. Brandt, 'The Hopkins Verbal Learning Test: Development of a new memory test with six equivalent forms', *Clinical Neuropsychologist*, vol. 5, no. 2, pp. 125–42, 1991.

M.F. Folstein et al., '"Mini-mental state". A practical method for grading the cognitive state of patients for the clinician', *Journal of Psychiatric Research*, vol. 12, no. 3, pp. 189–98, 1975.

D. LoGiudice et al., 'Kimberley Indigenous Cognitive Assessment tool (KICA): Development of a cognitive assessment tool for older Indigenous Australians', *International Psychogeriatrics*, vol. 18, no. 2, pp. 269–80, 2006.

Z.S. Nasreddine et al., 'The Montreal Cognitive Assessment, MoCA: A brief screening tool for mild cognitive impairment', *Journal of the American Geriatrics Society*, vol. 53, no. 4, pp. 695–69, 2005.

J.E. Storey et al., 'The Rowland Universal Dementia Assessment Scale

(RUDAS): A multicultural cognitive assessment scale', *International Psychogeriatrics*, vol. 16, no. 1, pp. 13–31, 2004.

Chapter 13: Investigations

R. Laforce et al., 'Molecular imaging in dementia: Past, present, and future', *Alzheimer's & Dementia*, vol. 14, no. 11, pp. 1522–52, 2018.

Chapter 15: Management of Cognitive Loss

Alzheimer's Society, 'Alcohol and dementia', 2020, www.alzheimers.org. uk/about-dementia/risk-factors-and-prevention/alcohol.

Better Health Channel, 'Alcohol related brain impairment – memory loss', 2015, www.betterhealth.vic.gov.au/health/conditionsandtreatments/ alcohol-related-brain-impairment-memory-loss.

K. Cherry, 'Does drinking alcohol kill brain cells?', *Very Well Mind*, 16 May 2020, www.verywellmind.com/does-drinking-alcohol-really-kill-brain-cells-2794887.

E.W. Dolan, 'Problematic alcohol use linked to reduced hippocampal volume', *PsyPost*, 9 December 2017, www.psypost.org/2017/12/ problematic-alcohol-use-linked-reduced-hippocampal-volume-50354.

I. McKeith et al., 'Neuroleptic sensitivity in patients with senile dementia of the Lewy body type', *British Medical Journal*, vol. 305, pp. 673–8, 1992.

R. McShane et al., 'Memantine for dementia', *The Cochrane Database of Systematic Reviews*, issue 3, article no. CD003154, 2019.

Medline Plus, 'Wernicke-Korsakoff syndrome', 2020, https://medlineplus. gov/ency/article/000771.htm.

M.F. Mendez et al., 'Preliminary findings: Behavioral worsening on donepezil in patients with frontotemporal dementia', *American Journal of Geriatric Psychiatry*, vol. 15, pp. 84–7, 2007.

National Health and Medical Research Council, *Draft Australian Guidelines to Reduce Health Risks from Drinking Alcohol*, December 2019, www. nhmrc.gov.au/sites/default/files/documents/attachments/draft-aus-guidelines-reduce-health-risks-alcohol.pdf.

D.W. Oslin & M.S. Cary, 'Alcohol-related dementia: Validation of diagnostic criteria', *American Journal of Geriatric Psychiatry*, vol. 11, no. 4, pp. 441–7, 2003.

N.J. Ridley et al., 'Alcohol-related dementia: An update of the evidence', *Alzheimer's Research & Therapy*, vol. 5, no. 1, p. 3, 2013.

A. Sachdeva et al., 'Alcohol-related dementia and neurocognitive impairment: A review study', *International Journal of High Risk Behaviors & Addiction*, vol. 5, no. 3, 2016.

R.H. Shmerling, 'Sorting out the health effects of alcohol', *Harvard Health Publishing*, 7 August 2018, www.health.harvard.edu/blog/sorting-out-the-health-effects-of-alcohol-2018080614427.

K.J. Woodburn & E.C. Johnstone, 'Early-onset dementia in Lothian, Scotland: An analysis of clinical features and patterns of decline', *Health Bulletin*, vol. 57, no. 6, pp. 384–92, 1999.

W. Xu et al., 'Alcohol consumption and dementia risk: A dose-response meta-analysis of prospective studies', *European Journal of Epidemiology*, vol. 32, no. 1, pp. 31–42, 2017.

Chapter 16: Behavioural and Psychological Symptoms of Dementia

G.S. Alexopoulos, 'The Cornell Scale for Depression in Dementia: Administration and scoring guidelines', Cornell Institute of Geriatric Psychiatry, 2012, www.scalesandmeasures.net/files/files/The%20Cornell%20Scale%20for%20Depression%20in%20Dementia.pdf.

S. Baillon et al., 'Valproate preparations for agitation in dementia', *The Cochrane Database of Systematic Reviews*, issue 10, article no. CD003945, 2018.

K.C. Buckwalter, 'Individualized plan of care based on Progressively Lowered Stress Threshold (PLST) model (Buckwalter)', Rosalynn Carter Institute for Caregiving, 2020, www.rosalynncarter.org/research/caregiver-intervention-database/individualized-plan-of-care-based-on-progressively-lowered-stress-threshold-plst-model-buckwalter.

J. Cohen-Mansfield, 'Theoretical frameworks for behavioural problems in dementia', *Alzheimer's Care Quarterly*, vol. 1, pp. 8–21, 2000.

N. Drouillard et al., 'Therapeutic approaches in the management of behavioral and psychological symptoms of dementia in the elderly', *BC Medical Journal*, vol. 55, no. 2, pp. 90–5, 2013.

S.L. Filan & R.H. Llewellyn-Jones, 'Animal-assisted therapy for dementia: A review of the literature', *International Psychogeriatrics*, vol. 18, no. 4, pp. 597–611, 2006.

S. Finkel, 'Introduction to behavioural and psychological symptoms of dementia (BPSD)', *International Journal of Geriatric Psychiatry*, vol. 15, no. S1, pp. 2–4, 2000.

J.E. Fisher et al., 'A contextual model of restraint–free care for persons with dementia', in P. Sturmey (ed.), *Functional Analysis in Clinical Treatment*, London, Elsevier, pp. 211–38, 2007.

G.R. Hall & K.C. Buckwalter, 'Progressively lowered stress threshold: A conceptual model for care of adults with Alzheimer's disease', *Archives of Psychiatric Nursing*, vol. 1, pp. 399–406, 1987.

S.L. Harrison et al., 'The dispensing of psychotropic medicines to older people before and after they enter residential aged care', *Medical Journal of Australia*, vol. 212, no. 7, pp. 309–13, 2020.

International Psychogeriatric Association, *IPA Complete Guides to Behavioral and Psychological Symptoms of Dementia (BPSD)*, fourth edition, 2012.

J.T. Olin et al., 'A pilot randomized trial of carbamazepine for behavioral symptoms in treatment-resistant outpatients with Alzheimer disease', *The American Journal of Geriatric Psychiatry*, vol. 9, no. 4, pp. 400–5, 2001.

R. Rea et al., 'Apathy in Alzheimer's disease: Any effective treatment?', *The Scientific World Journal*, vol. 2014, article no. 421,385, 2014.

N.E. Richeson, 'Effects of animal-assisted therapy on agitated behaviors and social interactions of older adults with dementia', *American Journal of Alzheimer's Disease & Other Dementias*, vol. 18, no. 6, pp. 353–8, 2003.

Royal Australian & New Zealand College of Psychiatrists, 'Antipsychotic medications as a treatment of behavioural and psychological symptoms of dementia' (fact sheet), August 2016, www.ranzcp.org/files/resources/college_statements/practice_guidelines/pg10-pdf.aspx.

J. Swearer, 'Behavioral disturbances in dementia', in J.C. Morris (ed), *Handbook of Dementing Illnesses*, New York, Marcel Dekker Inc., 1994.

P.N. Tariot et al., 'Efficacy and tolerability of carbamazepine for agitation and aggression in dementia', *The American Journal of Psychiatry*, vol. 155, no. 1, pp. 54–61, 1998.

O.P. Tible et al., 'Best practice in the management of behavioural and psychological symptoms of dementia', *Therapeutic Advances in Neurological Disorders*, vol. 10, no. 8, pp. 297–309, 2017.

R.E. Wragg & D.V. Jeste, 'Overview of depression and psychosis in Alzheimer's disease', *The American Journal of Psychiatry*, vol. 146, no. 5, pp. 577–87, 1989.

A. Yusupov & J.E. Galvin, 'Vocalization in dementia: A case report and review of the literature', *Case Reports in Neurology*, vol. 6, no. 1, pp. 126–33, 2014.

Chapter 17: Sleeping, Eating and Mobility

H.G. Bloom et al., 'Evidence-based recommendations for the assessment and management of sleep disorders in older persons', *Journal of the American Geriatric Society*, vol. 57, no. 5, pp. 761–89, 2009.

B. Broers et al., 'Prescription of a THC/CBD-based medication to patients with dementia: A pilot study in Geneva', *Medical Cannabis and Cannabinoids*, vol. 2, pp. 56–9, 2019.

P. Cullen et al., 'Eating disorders in dementia', *International Journal of Geriatric Psychiatry*, vol. 12, no. 5, pp. 559–62, 1997.

Dementia Australia, 'Meal times provide us with an opportunity to spend time with our family and friends, as well as sharing food together', 2020, www.dementia.org.au/information/about-you/i-am-a-carer-family-member-or-friend/personal-care/eating.

K.A. Josephs et al., 'Coprophagia in neurologic disorders', *Journal of Neurology*, vol. 263, no. 5, p. 1008, 2016.

K.M. Kinnunen et al., 'The management of sleep disorders in dementia', *Current Opinion in Psychiatry*, vol. 30, no. 6, pp. 491–7, 2017.

O. Piguet et al., 'Sensitivity of current criteria for the diagnosis of behavioral variant frontotemporal dementia', *Neurology*, vol. 72, no. 8, pp. 732–7, 2009.

K.M. Rose & R. Lorenz, 'Sleep disturbances in dementia', *Journal of Gerontological Nursing*, vol. 36, no. 5, pp. 9–14, 2010.

M.B. Sandilyan, 'Abnormal eating patterns in dementia – a cause for concern', *Age and Ageing*, vol. 40, eLetters Supplement, November 2011.

C.H. Schenck et al., 'Delayed emergence of a parkinsonian disorder or dementia in 81% of older men initially diagnosed with idiopathic rapid eye movement sleep behavior disorder: A 16-year update on a previously reported series', *Sleep Medicine*, vol. 14, no. 8, pp. 744–8, 2013.

SleepFoundation.org, 'Sleep hygiene', 29 July 2020, www.sleepfoundation.org/articles/sleep-hygiene.

M.I. Tolea et al., 'Trajectory of mobility decline by type of dementia', *Alzheimer Disease and Associated Disorders*, vol. 30, no. 1, pp. 60–6, 2016.

M. Walker, *Why We Sleep: The new science of sleep and dreams*, Penguin Press, 2018.

Chapter 18: Continence, Urinary Tract Infections and Sexuality

Alzheimer Society of Canada, 'Conversations about dementia, intimacy and sexuality' (fact sheet), 2018, https://alzheimer.ca/sites/default/files/files/national/brochures-conversations/conversations_intimacy-and-sexuality.pdf.

B. Black et al., 'Inappropriate sexual behaviors in dementia', *Journal of Geriatric Psychiatry and Neurology*, vol. 18, no. 3, pp. 155–62, 2005.

Continence Foundation of Australia, 'Dementia', 2020, www.continence.org.au/pages/dementia.html.

R.G. Jepson et al., 'Cranberries for preventing urinary tract infections', *The Cochrane Database of Systematic Reviews*, issue 10, article no. CD001321, 2012.

W. Marsiglio & D. Donnelly, 'Sexual relations in later life: A national study of married persons', *Journal of Gerontology*, vol. 46, pp. S338–S344, 1991.

K. Panesar, 'Drug-induced urinary incontinence', *U.S. Pharmacist*, 20 August 2014, www.uspharmacist.com/article/druginduced-urinary-incontinence.

B.D. Starr & M.B. Weiner, *The Starr-Weiner Report on Sex and Sexuality in Mature Years*, New York, McGraw-Hill, 1981.

P. Yap & D. Tan, 'Urinary incontinence in dementia – a practical approach', *Australian Family Physician*, vol. 35, no. 4, pp. 237–41, 2006.

Chapter 19: Pain and Skin Integrity

J. Abbey et al., 'The Abbey pain scale: A 1-minute numerical indicator for people with end-stage dementia', *International Journal of Palliative Nursing*, vol. 10, no. 1, pp. 6–13, 2004.

Faculty of Pain Medicine of the Royal College of Anaesthetists, 'Dose equivalents and changing opioids', n.d., https://fpm.ac.uk/opioids-aware-structured-approach-opioid-prescribing/dose-equivalents-and-changing-opioids.

J.C. Huffman & M.E. Kunik, 'Assessment and understanding of pain in patients with dementia', *Gerontologist*, vol. 40, pp. 574–81, 2000.

C.J. Maxwell et al., 'The prevalence and management of current daily pain among older home care clients', *Pain*, vol. 138, pp. 208–16, 2008.

Park, H., 'Effect of music on pain for home-dwelling persons with dementia', *Pain Management Nursing*, vol. 11, pp. 141–7, 2010.

SA Health, 'Adverse effects due to long term opioids' (fact sheet), n.d., www.sahealth.sa.gov.au/wps/wcm/connect/1dc75100499f9ab280 f2de9b6ca12d15/Fact+sheet.adverse+effects+due+to+longterm+ opioids.patients.pdf.

J.W. Shega et al., 'Pain in community-dwelling persons with dementia: Frequency, intensity, and congruence between patient and caregiver report', *Journal of Pain Symptoms Management*, vol. 28, pp. 585–92, 2004.

Chapter 20: Communication

Alzheimer's Society, 'Tips: Communicating with someone with dementia', 2020, www.alzheimers.org.uk/about-dementia/symptoms-and-diagnosis/symptoms/tips-for-communicating-dementia.

C. McCabe & F. Timmins, *Communication Skills for Nursing Practice*, second edition, Red Globe Press, 2013.

F. Sugden-Best, *Sourcebook for Assessing & Maintaining Communication*, Speechmark Publishing Ltd, quoted in D. Jootun & G. McGhee, 'Effective communication with people who have dementia', *Nursing Standard*, vol. 25, no. 25, pp. 40–6, 23 February 2011.

Chapter 21: Legal Issues and Advanced Care Planning

Advance Care Planning Australia (website), www.advancecareplanning.org.au.

Dementia Australia, 'Dementia and driving', 2020, www.dementia.org.au/resources/dementia-and-driving.

Chapter 22: Ethics, Consent and Elder Abuse

Alzheimer's Association, 'Abuse', 2020, www.alz.org/help-support/caregiving/safety/abuse.

Australian Institute of Family Studies, 'What is known about the prevalence and dynamics of elder abuse', https://aifs.gov.au/publications/elder-abuse.

Elder Abuse Prevention Unit, 'Risk factors' (fact sheet), n.d., www.eapu.com.au/uploads/information/Fact%20Sheet%20-%20Risk%20Factors.docx.

T. Gracyk, 'Four fundamental ethical principles (a very simple introduction)', 2012, http://web.mnstate.edu/gracyk/courses/ phil%20115/Four_Basic_principles.htm.

Nuffield Council on Bioethics, *Dementia: Ethical issues*, 2009, http:// nuffieldbioethics.org/wp-content/uploads/2014/07/Dementia-short-guide.pdf.

Relationships Australia, 'What is elder abuse?', 2020, www.relationships.org. au/relationship-advice/relationship-advice-sheets/what-is-elder-abuse.

K.L. Smebye et al., 'Ethical dilemmas concerning autonomy when persons with dementia wish to live at home: A qualitative, hermeneutic study', *BMC Health Services Research*, vol. 16, no. 21, 2016.

P.J. Whitehouse, 'Ethical issues in dementia', *Dialogues in Clinical Neuroscience*, vol. 2, no. 2, pp. 162–7, 2000.

Chapter 23: Minimising Carer Stress and Obtaining Support

Australian Government, *My Aged Care* (website), www.myagedcare.gov.au.

International Psychogeriatric Association, *IPA Complete Guides to Behavioral and Psychological Symptoms of Dementia (BPSD)*, fourth edition, 2012.

Chapter 24: Entering Residential Care

Australian Government, *My Aged Care* (website), www.myagedcare.gov.au.

Dementia Australia, 'Deciding on residential care', 2020, www.dementia. org.au/support-and-services/families-and-friends/residential-care/ deciding-on-residential-care.

Chapter 25: Cultivating Happiness and Meaning in Dementia

Dementia Care Notes, 'Improve the quality of life of persons with dementia', 2020, https://dementiacarenotes.in/caregivers/quality-of-life.

R. Parsons, 'A caregiver's guide: Creating joy and meaning for those with dementia', *Alzheimers.net*, 15 May 2015, www.alzheimers.net/5-15-15-caregivers-guide-joy-and-meaning-for-dementia.

Chapter 26: Dying and End-of-life Care

Alzheimer's Australia, *End of Life Care for People with Dementia: Survey Report 2014: Executive Summary*, Alzheimer's Australia, 2014, www. dementia.org.au/sites/default/files/EOI_ExecSummary_Web_ Version.pdf.

Better Health Channel, 'Dealing with news about dying', Department of Health and Human Services, 2017, www.betterhealth.vic.gov.au/health/servicesandsupport/Dealing-with-news-about-dying.

Dementia Australia, 'Palliative care and dementia', Dementia Australia, paper number 43, 2017, https://palliativecare.org.au/wp-content/uploads/dlm_uploads/2018/05/Dementia-Aus-Palliative-Care-Discussion-Paper-36pp-R5.pdf.

C. Elton, 'Redefining dementia as a terminal illness', *Time*, 14 October 2009.

NSW Health, 'End-of-life care and decision-making – guidelines', Ministry of Health NSW, 2005, www1.health.nsw.gov.au/pds/ActivePDSDocuments/GL2005_057.pdf.

Index